BIOMEDICAL & NANOMEDICAL TECHNOLOGIES
CONCISE MONOGRAPH SERIES

Design of Mechanical Bearings in Cardiac Assist Devices

Said Jahanmir

Andrew Hunsberger

Hooshang Heshmat

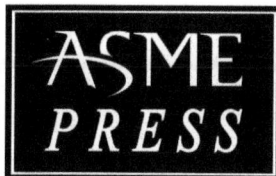

ASME
PRESS

Library of Congress Cataloging-in-Publication Data

Names: Jahanmir, Said. | Hunsberger, Andrew. | Heshmat, Hooshang. | American Society of Mechanical Engineers.
Title: Design of mechanical bearings in cardiac assist devices / Said Jahanmir, Andrew Hunsberger, and Hooshang Heshmat.
Description: New York : ASME Press, [2016] | "The American Society of Mechanical Engineers." | Includes bibliographical references.
Identifiers: LCCN 2016026673 | ISBN 9780791860427
Subjects: LCSH: Heart, Mechanical. | Bearings (Machinery)--Design and construction. | Biomedical engineering. | Pumping machinery.
Classification: LCC RD598.35.M42 J34 2016 | DDC 617.4/120592--dc23 LC record available at https://lccn.loc.gov/2016026673

Guest Editors' Preface

According to the American Heart Association, approximately 5 million Americans have congestive heart failure (CHF) and more than half a million new cases are reported every year. CHF is a chronic condition in which at least one chamber of the heart is not pumping well enough to meet the body's need. Heart failure presents an increasing public burden of morbidity and mortality even as the mortality from coronary artery disease and hypertension is decreasing. It is estimated that at least 40,000 of these patients are candidates for heart transplantation; however, only 3,800 donor hearts are made available each year worldwide. While effective pharmacologic therapies have improved outcomes for mild to moderate CHF, the need for mechanical circulatory support is well defined and growing.

Current use of mechanical circulatory cardiac devices is dominated by the indications of post-cardiotomy shock and bridging to transplantation. About 6,000 patients a year receive support devices after cardiac surgery, in the U.S. alone. However, most of the devices do not allow for hospital discharge of patients. If fully implantable and wearable devices were available, at least 100,000 patients annually could benefit from this technology.

Significant technological advances have been made in the past thirty years in the design and development of mechanical cardiac circulatory support devices. Several recent review articles and book chapters have summarized the state-of-the-art in this critical medical technology. However, a comprehensive and focused publication on this subject is currently lacking. The comprehensive review articles in this concise monograph series have been written by an international team of experts with many years of experience in design of mechanical cardiovascular assist devices and performance evaluation, both in pre-clinical and clinical testing, as well as issues related to standards and regulatory requirements.

Said Jahanmir
William J. Weiss
Conrad M. Zapanta

Series Editors' Preface

Biomedical and Nanomedical Technologies (B&NT)
This concise monograph series focuses on the implementation of various engineering principles in the conception, design, development, analysis and operation of biomedical, biotechnological and nanotechnology systems and applications. The primary objective of the series is to compile the latest research topics in biomedical and nanomedical technologies, specifically devices and materials.

Each volume comprises a collection of invited manuscripts, written in an accessible manner and of a concise and manageable length. These timely collections will provide an invaluable resource for initial enquiries about technologies, encapsulating the latest developments and applications with reference sources for further detailed information. The content and format have been specifically designed to stimulate further advances and applications of these technologies by reaching out to the non-specialist across a broad audience.

Contributions to *Biomedical and Nanomedical Technologies* will inspire interest in further research and development using these technologies and encourage other potential applications. This will foster the advancement of biomedical and nanomedical applications, ultimately improving healthcare delivery.

Editor:
Ahmed Al-Jumaily, PhD, Professor of Biomechanical Engineering & Director of the Institute of Biomedical Technologies, Auckland University of Technology.

Associate Editors:
Christopher H.M. Jenkins, PhD, PE, Professor and Head, Mechanical & Industrial Engineering Department, Montana State University.

Said Jahanmir, PhD, President & CEO, Boston Tribology Associates.

Shanzhong (Shawn) Duan, PhD, Professor, Mechanical Engineering, South Dakota State University.

Conrad M. Zapanta, PhD, Associate Department Head of Biomedical Engineering, Teaching Professor of Biomedical Engineering, Carnegie Mellon University.

William J. Weiss, PhD, Professor of Surgery and Bioengineering, College of Medicine, The Pennsylvania State University.

Contents

Abstract

Continuous flow, mechanical cardiac assist devices rely on a rotating impeller to aid the heart with blood flow. Like any other mechanical system, the rotating components of these devices require some form of load support that is provided by either mechanical or magnetic bearings. The goal of this article is to provide an overview of basic principles that are important for design and evaluation of mechanical bearings used in blood pumps with a primary focus on mechanical bearings used in the second and third generation ventricular assist devices (VADs). A general introduction of some basic principles that are important for design of mechanical bearings is first provided. The basic function of lubricants is described and a brief introduction is provided for surface roughness and the concept of real area of contact. Different lubrication regimes (boundary, mixed and fluid film) are defined. Rheological properties of different types of fluids are described. In the boundary lubrication regime contact lubrication is controlled by the physical and chemical properties of thin films, whereas in the hydrodynamic lubrication regime only physical and rheological properties of the thick fluid films are important. Principles of hydrodynamic lubrication are described and different types of fluid film bearings are discussed. Reynolds Equation which is the fundamental base for fluid film lubrication is discussed and its application to the design of different types of bearings is explored. An example for the design of a blood lubricated thrust bearing is provided. Lubrication of contact bearings is described and some challenging issues such as contact damage are briefly introduced. Boundary lubrication with molecular films is described. Fundamental mechanisms of wear and damage formation as well as the use of hard ceramic materials to combat wear are described. Finally examples are provided for current assist devices where blood lubricated contact bearings or hydrodynamic bearings are used.

1. Introduction

The goal of this article is to provide an overview of basic principles that are important for design and evaluation of bearings used in blood pumps. While the primary focus is on mechanical bearings used in the second and third generation ventricular assist devices (VADs), bearings used in the first generation pulsatile devices as well as those used in percutaneous and extracorporeal applications are also described. The new generation of continuous flow VADs uses rotating impellers to accelerate the blood and increase the fluid pressure while delivering the required flow rate. These rotary pumps are classified as either axial or centrifugal flow devices. In the axial flow pumps, the fluid, in this case blood, enters at one end of the cylindrical pump housing, follows the axial direction of the housing, and exits at the other end. In contrast with this flow geometry, the impellers used in centrifugal pumps push the fluid out of the housing in the radial direction. In either case, the rotating impeller requires load support in the axial and the radial directions. This support mechanism is provided either by magnetic bearings or by blood-lubricated mechanical bearings.

The schematic in Figure 1-1a shows a simplified geometry of an axial pump, with the flow entering from the left and exiting from the right in the axial direction. Radial support is needed to maintain the radial position of the rotating group that may include the impeller and the motor elements. Axial support is needed to counter the force of fluid entering the pump. A similar set of journal (radial support) and thrust (axial support) bearings are required in a centrifugal pump shown in Figure 1-1b. In this case the flow enters in the axial direction and exits in the radial direction. Different bearing configurations can be used and in general include contact and fluid-lubricated bearings.

Direct mechanical contact is made between the two surfaces in contact bearings, often with a molecularly thin lubricant film at the interface. A popular and practical contact bearing is the pivot bearing, shown in Figure 1-2a. This is commonly known as the jewel bearing and has been used in mechanical watches for many years [1]. A sapphire or diamond jewel is usually used against a high strength steel pivot, often cylindrical or conical with a hemispherical end. The recess in the jewel is also hemispherical. Both components must be highly polished

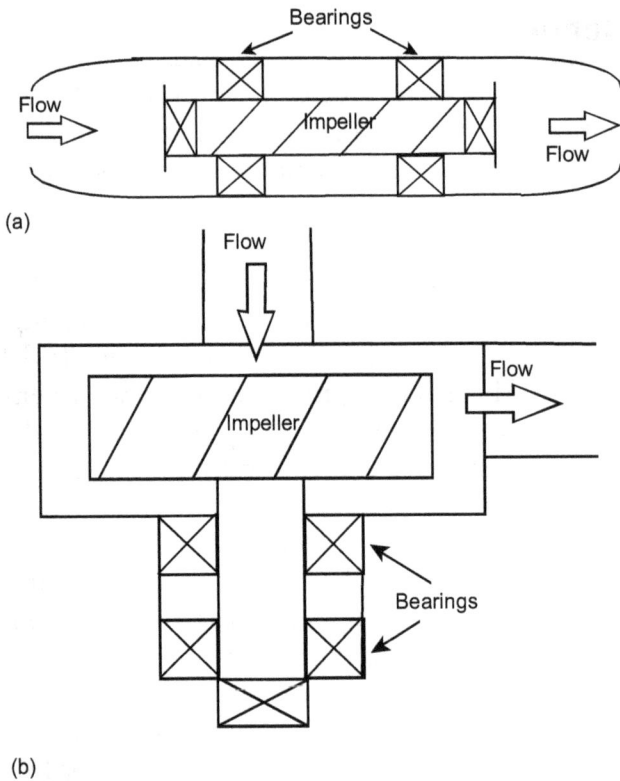

Figure 1-1 Typical design of blood pumps, with bearings providing axial and radial support shown by the rectangular boxes: (a) axial flow pump with fluid entering from the right and exiting to the left and (b) centrifugal pump with fluid entering from the top and exiting to the right.

and fabricated to close dimensional tolerances for best performance. In special cases, a spherical ball is used with two jewels instead of a single cylindrical pivot, Figure 1-2b. Pivot bearings provide axial load support during rotation of either the pivot or the jewel, but they cannot provide radial support. Possible locations for such bearings in axial pumps are at both ends of the impeller, Figure 1-1a; and in centrifugal flow pumps they are located below the impeller, Figure 1-1b, to support the impeller against the force of the flowing blood. These bearings are usually immersed in blood, and a thin fluid film migrates in between the surfaces and provides boundary lubrication (defined in Sections 1.1 and 3.2).

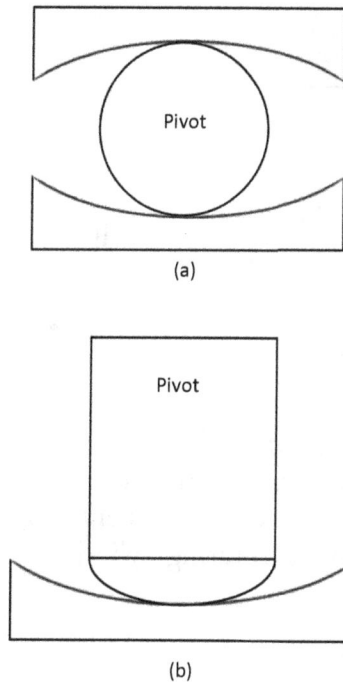

Figure 1-2 Typical pivot bearings: (a) Jewel bearing with a hemispherical ended pivot, (b) Bearing with a spherical pivot and two jewels.

In contrast with the pivot bearings, fluid-lubricated bearings are designed to provide either radial or axial support or a combination of both. While the two components of the pivot bearing are either in intimate contact or separated by a thin fluid film, the components in a fluid-lubricated bearing are separated by a relatively thick film of fluid, as shown in Figure 1-3a and b for thrust and journal bearings. The lubricant film, and therefore load support, is developed due to the movement of the fluid into the gap between the moving surfaces. Since the fluid film is developed by the hydrodynamic forces as a result of the fluid being forced into the gap, it is important to note that the surfaces in these bearings are in contact before the start of rotation and after the rotation ceases. The design and performance of these hydrodynamically lubricated bearings are described in Section 2 following a brief discussion on characteristics of surfaces, lubrication regimes and rheological properties of fluids.

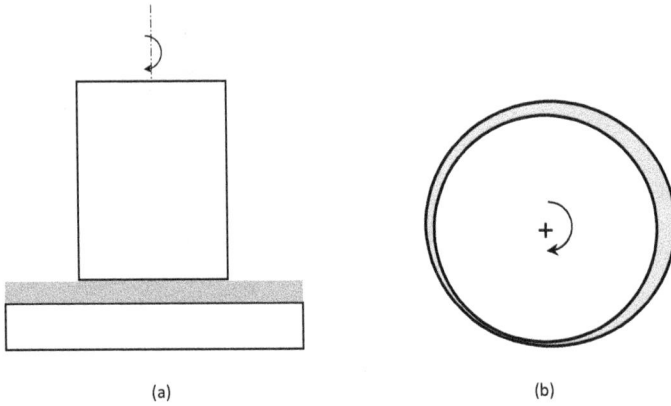

(a) (b)

Figure 1-3 Typical fluid lubricated bearings: (a) Thrust bearing with the upper cylindrical component rotating and the stationary flat lower component, (b) Journal bearing composed of a loaded rotating cylinder inside a cylindrical bushing.

1.1 Characteristics of surfaces

In order to assess the physics and chemistry of contacting surfaces it is instructive to first review the structure and chemical properties of solid surfaces. All solid surfaces possess certain geometric patterns that are characteristic of the manufacturing process used to prepare the surface. For example, a surface created by machining, such as milling or turning, would have a series of roughly parallel machining marks, visible to the naked eye. If such a surface is viewed at a higher magnification, smaller perturbations would become evident in addition to the machining marks, as shown in the surface profile in Figure 1-4a. In comparison with the regular profile generated by turning, surfaces prepared by grinding have more random features, Figure 1-4b. These surface profiles have been obtained with a conventional profilometer, which records the traces made by a diamond stylus as it traverses across the surface. Note that in both cases the vertical magnification is at least 100 times larger than the horizontal scale. Therefore, the surface is not as ragged as the profile traces show. In general the average slope of surface features is about 2-5 degrees. Surface profiles are used to calculate various statistical parameters such roughness average R_a, rms (root mean square) roughness R_q, mean peak spacing S_m, skewness R_{sk}, and others [2].

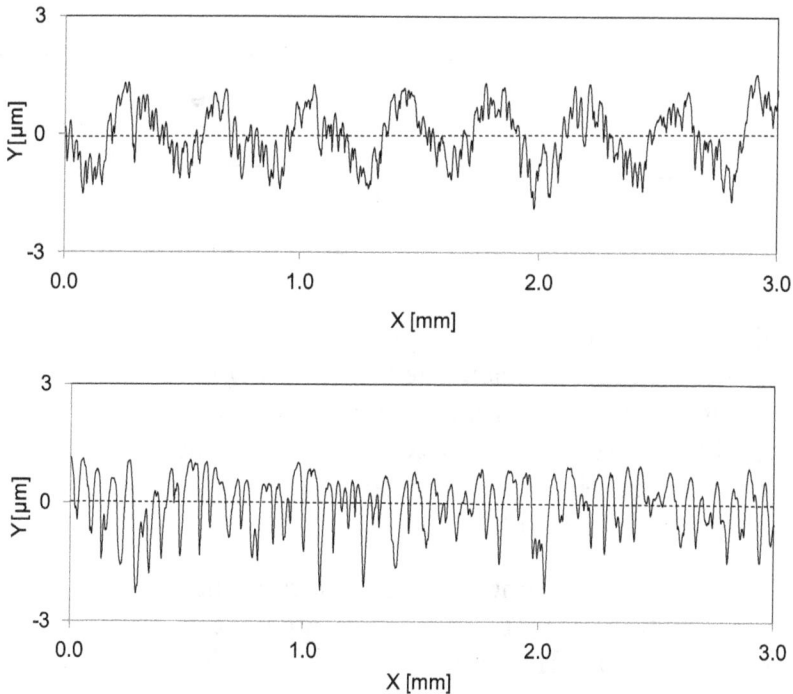

Figure 1-4 Typical surface roughness for surfaces prepared by turning (a) and grinding (b) with the same surface roughness Ra = 0.56 μm.

These statistical values, taken together, can describe the profile of a particular surface. Such descriptions of the profiles are very important when two surfaces are brought into contact.

Practically all metals except gold are covered by thin oxide layers that protect the surfaces against further oxidation. The outermost layer on top of the oxide layer will contain adsorbed species from the environment, such as oxygen, nitrogen, carbon, moisture and others. The surface could contain hydrocarbon species for example from contact with human skin or oils from fabrication processes. In addition to metals, non-oxide ceramics also have thin naturally grown oxide layers. The oxide layers and adsorbed compounds often play important roles in tribological properties of surfaces in contact [3].

When two surfaces are pressed together under normal load, the actual contact occurs between the uppermost asperities, Figure 1-5a.

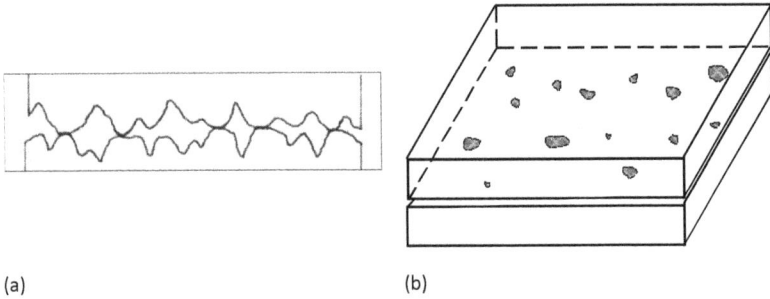

(a)   (b)

Figure 1-5 Real area of contact when two rough surfaces are brought into contact. The 2-D drawing in (a) shows five contact points, and (b) shows distribution of real area of contact in 3-D. The size of the contact patches can range from a few to several tens of micrometers depending on the contacting materials and load.

Summation of asperity contact areas constitutes the real area of contact, which is usually 1/10 to 1/1000 of the apparent or geometric area of contact, Figure 1-5b. The actual normal load is then taken up only on the asperity contacts and not the entire apparent area. The physical and chemical processes associated with the highly loaded asperity contacts give rise to complex set of events when the surfaces are in relative sliding motion against each other. The measured friction force between the two sliding surfaces and the observed surface damage or wear are the result of mechanical and chemical interactions at the asperities. Strong interatomic attractions (adhesion forces) occur giving rise to the friction force when one surface is slid against another under a normal load. Combination of normal and tangential forces acting on the asperity contacts can result in deformation and fracture of the contacts giving rise to the generation of wear particles. Heat dissipated as the frictional energy is expended. Combination of thermal interactions and mechanical deformation produces non-equilibrium chemical reactions between the contacting surfaces and any other species in the surrounding area (i.e., the lubricant, or air). These processes are often referred to as tribochemical interactions and produce solid surface layers with complex chemical and physical structures. Often formation and removal of such chemically complex products control the wear process of two sliding surfaces, making it difficult, if not impossible to fully understand the fundamentals that control the friction and wear processes [3].

1.2 Lubrication regimes

High friction between two sliding surfaces, for example metals, produces high levels of surface damage and a high rate of wear. Therefore, it is necessary to protect the surfaces with some form of lubrication. A lubricant, by definition, is any substance that modifies the friction and/or wear performance of contacting surfaces. As such any material - gas, fluid, or solid – that reduces friction is considered as a lubricant. However, a good lubricant must also possess other attributes such as corrosion resistance, stability, durability, etc. When fluids are used as lubricants to protect sliding surfaces, two fundamental lubrication regimes are observed: boundary lubrication and fluid film lubrication. In highly loaded contacts at low sliding speeds with low viscosity fluids, the two bodies remain in intimate contact with only a thin molecular film in between. The term "boundary lubrication" is used to describe this lubrication regime. However, when a thicker lubricant film is developed during high speed sliding of lightly loaded surfaces lubricated with higher viscosity fluids, the term "hydrodynamic lubrication" or fluid film lubrication is used. The two lubrication regimes are depicted in Figure 1-6, which also shows an intermediate regime, or "mixed lubrication", where

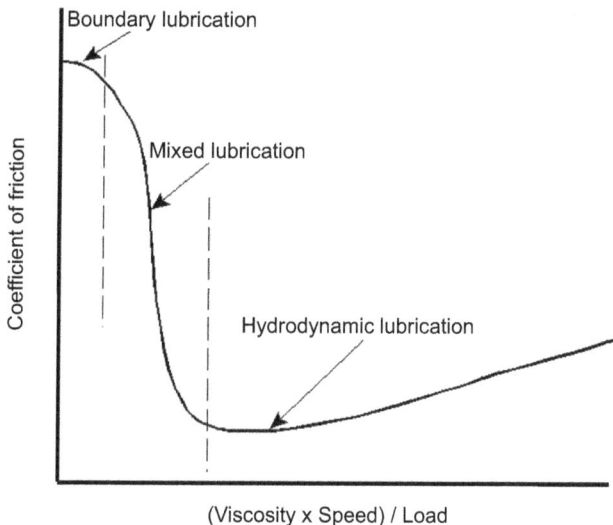

Figure 1-6 Stribeck lubrication curve showing three lubrication regimes: Boundary lubrication, Mixed lubrication and Hydrodynamic lubrication. Adopted from reference [4].

both boundary and thick film lubrication regimes are concurrently active. The figure is based on experimental work of Stribeck [4] and plots the coefficient of friction (tangential force/normal force) against the product of viscosity and sliding velocity divided by normal load. The friction coefficient in the boundary lubrication regime generally ranges from 0.01 to 0.2 and is on the order of 0.001 in the fluid film regime. Note that in the hydrodynamic lubrication regime the lubricant film thickness is much larger than the roughness height (generally at least 3 times larger).

In the mixed lubrication regime the relative film thickness increases and the surfaces are pushed apart due to hydrodynamic effects. The friction coefficient decreases as the influence of boundary lubrication is diminished and the fluid film lubrication becomes more dominant. The friction and wear performance of lubricated systems are controlled by a complex interplay between physical and chemical properties of surfaces and the lubricant in the boundary regime. However, in the fluid film regime only the physical properties of the lubricant, i.e., the rheological properties, control the lubrication behavior. In this lubrication regime, the friction coefficient increases due to increased fluid shear as a result of increased viscosity or speed.

1.3 Rheological properties of fluids

Viscosity is an important rheological property of fluids that determines its flow characteristics in narrow gaps such as in bearings. Viscosity is the measure of fluid's resistance to flow when subjected to shear stress. According to Newton's law of viscous flow the shear stress is proportional to the rate of change of velocity with respect to the film height

$$\tau = \eta \frac{du}{dy} \qquad (1\text{-}1)$$

where η is the fluid viscosity and du/dy is the velocity gradient or the shear rate (see Figure 1-7). If it is assumed that the shear rate is constant, then

$$\tau = \eta \frac{U}{h} \qquad (1\text{-}2)$$

Many simple liquids, such as water, glycerol and mineral oils follow this simple linear relationship such that the viscosity is independent of shear rate and time. These fluids are considered as Newtonian fluids.

However, many other fluids such as blood, polymer solutions, suspensions, emulsions and greases, and also simple fluids at high shear rates, do not follow the linear relationship and are considered as non-Newtonian fluids. A comparison between Newtonian and a few types of non-Newtonian behaviors are shown in Figure 1-7. The viscosity for a Newtonian fluid is independent of shear rate, as already stated. In this case, viscosity, or the slope of shear stress vs. shear rate is constant. For other fluids, viscosity varies with shear rate or time. For example, viscosity increases with shear rate in dilatants fluids. These fluids are considered as shear thickening fluids; examples include very concentrated suspensions. In contrast with this behavior, the viscosity of pseudoplastic fluids decreases as the shear rate is increased. Examples of these shear thinning fluids include polymeric solutions. Another example of non-Newtonian fluids is the Bingham solid, which will behave as a solid and does not flow until shear stress reaches a critical yield value. Very thick fluids such as greases follow this behavior. While Newtonian fluids are amenable to simplified flow analyses, full evaluation of non-Newtonian fluids are complex. Therefore, in many instances analysis of flow in bearings and bearing design starts with the assumption of the fluid being a simple Newtonian fluid. This, however, can introduce

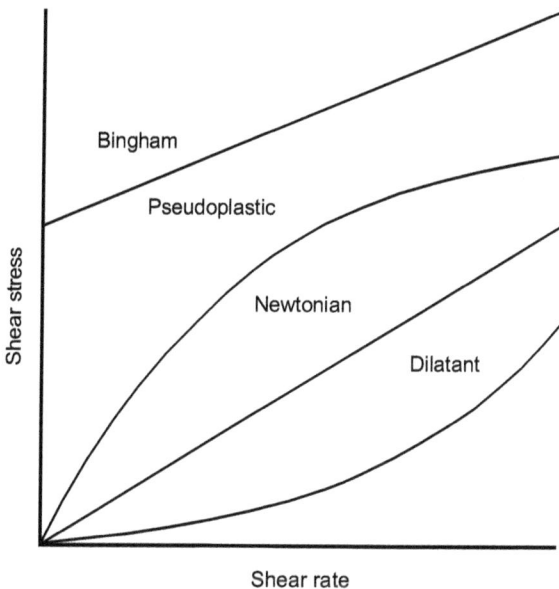

Figure 1-7   Rheological properties of different fluid types.

serious errors and divergence from experimental results obtained with the real non-Newtonian fluids.

Blood is composed of plasma and several types of cells (particles) such as erythrocytes (red blood cells), leukocytes (white blood cells) and thrombocytes (platelets). While plasma can be considered as a Newtonian fluid, whole blood (plasma and cells) exhibits a non-Newtonian shear thinning pseudoplastic behavior. This is related to the fact that red blood cells become oriented in the direction of flow as the shear rate or velocity increases. This effect becomes more pronounced in small blood vessels and small gaps, for example in blood pump bearings. *Therefore, caution should be exercised when whole blood is assumed to be a Newtonian fluid during analysis and design of blood lubricated bearings.*

2. Hydrodynamic lubrication

As indicated in Figure 1-3, there are two types of bearing configurations: (1) thrust bearing to support the normal load and (2) journal bearing to support the radial load. Often separate thrust and journal bearings are designed and implemented to support a rotating impeller. In certain cases more complex designs are used to combine the two bearing types. Nevertheless, the basic geometry that makes load support possible in hydrodynamic bearings is a converging wedge. In other words, the fluid is pulled into a converging gap through shear and a force perpendicular to the flow direction is produced, providing load support. Analysis of flow and prediction of load carrying ability of bearings starts with the Reynolds equation.

2.1 Reynolds equation

The Reynolds equation is a differential equation that describes the generation of hydrodynamic pressure within the lubricant film based on velocities of the solid surfaces, shape of the fluid film (or gap between the surfaces) and physical properties of the lubricant.

$$\frac{1}{6}\left\{ \frac{\partial}{\partial x}\left(\frac{h^3}{\eta}\cdot\frac{\partial p}{\partial x}\right) + \frac{\partial}{\partial z}\left(\frac{h^3}{\eta}\cdot\frac{\partial p}{\partial z}\right) \right\} = \left(v_o - v_1 \right)\frac{\partial h}{\partial x} + h\frac{\partial(v_o + v_1)}{\partial x} + 2\frac{\partial h}{\partial t}$$

$$(2\text{-}1)$$

Where p is the pressure developed due to the converging gap, η is the fluid viscosity, h is the fluid film thickness, and v_0 and v_1 are velocities of the two surfaces. The Reynolds equation neglects the inertial effects since they are generally much smaller than the viscous forces. It is also assumed that the fluid is Newtonian, has a constant viscosity and is incompressible. Lubricant film thickness is assumed to be small compared to the geometric dimensions of the bearing, and the fluid is assumed to adhere to the solid boundary, i.e., no slip between the fluid and bearing surfaces. Also, surface tension effects are neglected. These simplifying assumptions allow for pressure and flow evaluations for most common bearing problems. However, advanced analyses have been performed for complex bearing problems that require changes to the above assumptions [5]. These special cases are beyond the scope of this article.

The right side of the Reynolds equation contains three terms each with a different physical significance. These are referred to as the wedge, stretch, and squeeze contributions to load support. The first wedge term is the most important of the three, particularly with respect to common hydrodynamic bearings. It includes the contribution of the shape of the fluid film, $\partial h/\partial x$ (i.e., the converging wedge) and the relative velocity of the two surfaces, $(v_0 - v_1)$. The second stretch term is negligible, except for elastomeric bearings or special cases of dynamically loaded bearings. This term includes the contribution of pressure changes due to velocity variations in the sliding direction, for example due to stretching (or elastic deformation) of the bearing surfaces. The third squeeze contribution is due to normal approach of the surfaces, for example by impact, slow speed squeeze action, or relative normal vibrations [6].

For illustrative purposes, a converging wedge is shown in Figure 2-1. In this case the upper surface is stationary ($v_0 = 0$) and the lower surface moves in the x-direction at constant velocity $v_1 = U$. The bearing length in the x-direction is B. Fluid is drawn into the gap in the positive x-direction. The gap height h is a function of x and varies from entrance (h_i) to exit (h_o). Neglecting the stretch and squeeze effects, the Reynolds equation in one dimension for this problem is reduced to:

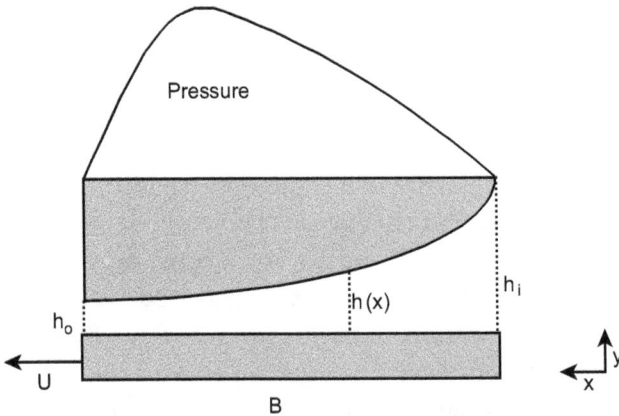

Figure 2-1 A hydrodynamically lubricated curved bearing. The upper surface is stationary and the lower surface with a length B moves to the left with speed U. The lubricant is drawn into the gap from right to left. Pressure distribution generated by the flow entering the bearing gap h is shown on top of the upper surface.

$$\frac{dp}{dx} = 6\eta U \frac{h - \bar{h}}{h^3} \qquad (2\text{-}2)$$

Note that $\bar{h}$ is the film thickness at the location of maximum pressure where $dp/dx = 0$. This is an elementary but useful form of Reynolds equation in one dimension. Integration of this equation for a given film shape, i.e., $h(x)$ provides the pressure distribution. Then, a second integration over the bearing area results in the bearing load. Inspection of this equation demonstrates that pressure variation depends on the viscosity and speed, in addition to the film thickness and shape. Pressure increases as the viscosity or the speed is increased and the film thickness is reduced.

2.2 Thrust bearing configurations

The most common and simplest geometry for a hydrodynamic bearing is the plane tapered configuration with a constant slope, shown in Figure 2-2a. Solution for the case shown would indicate that load carrying ability of the bearing is sensitive to the film thickness ratio ($H = h_i/h_o$); the larger the ratio of inlet to outlet film thickness, the larger is the load capacity. The tapered land bearing, however, is not practical for most applications. As the sliding stops, the load carrying capacity is reduced to zero and the sharp bearing edge will make contact with the counterface, causing surface damage and wear. A modified version is shown in Figure 2-2b, where a flat region is added to the tapered section. This plane tapered land configuration is widely used for thrust bearings. Another variation which is simpler to fabricate is the step bearing shown in Figure 2-2c. Note that the maximum pressure occurs near the minimum gap for the tapered and tapered land bearings, and at the step for the step bearing.

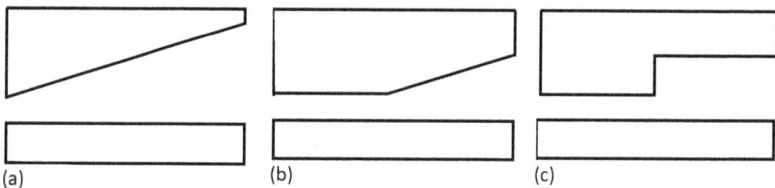

(a) (b) (c)

Figure 2-2 Simple thrust bearings: (a) tapered, (b) tapered land, and (c) step bearing.

If we define a non-dimensional load parameter W^* as

$$W^* = \frac{W h_0^2}{U \eta L B^2} \tag{2-3}$$

solution of the one dimensional Reynolds equation for the load carrying capacity of a simple tapered bearing in Figure 2-2a reduces to:

$$W^* = \frac{6}{H-1}\left(\frac{\ln H}{H-1} - \frac{2}{H+1}\right) \tag{2-4}$$

where W is the total load carried by the bearing, L and B are the dimensions in the z and x directions and H is the film thickness ratio

$$H = \frac{h_i}{h_o} \tag{2-5}$$

The relationship between W^* and H is graphically shown in Figure 2-3. The non-dimensional load parameter is at its maximum value of 0.16 when the film thickness ratio is equal to 2.3. These values are slightly modified for the tapered land bearing. It can be shown that the optimum configuration, i.e., maximum load capacity ($W^* = 0.192$), for the tapered land bearing occurs when the ratio of the ramp length to the total bearing length is equal to 0.8 and the film thickness ratio $H = 2.25$.

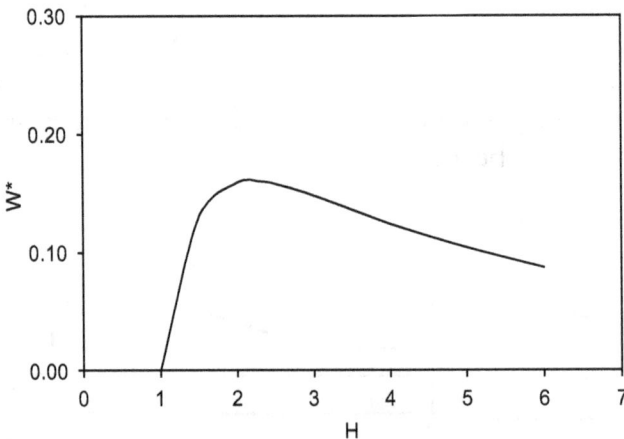

Figure 2-3   Non-dimensional load parameter versus film thickness ratio for an infinitely wide tapered bearing [6].

Therefore, the tapered land bearing provides a higher load capacity than a comparable tapered bearing.

The analyses for simple one dimensional bearing geometries discussed so far illustrate the importance of some of the geometric parameters. Actual bearings are more complex and the Reynolds equation can be extended for the analysis of two-dimensional bearings such as the tapered land thrust bearing shown in Figure 2-4. It should be noted that in such bearings not all of the fluid goes through the bearing, and a significant amount of the fluid leaks out from the sides. The geometry of a single pad is shown in Figure 2-5. The pad is characterized by an extent in the radial direction as B, width L, radius R, and the sector angle β. In cross-section, this is a tapered land bearing, with the extent of the flat region designated as D, where $D/B = \lambda$. The normalized load per pad for this configuration is defined as

$$W^* = \frac{W/L}{\omega \eta R}\left(\frac{h_o}{R\beta}\right)^2 \qquad (2\text{-}6)$$

Note that this relation is similar to Equation 2-3 for an infinite one dimensional bearing, where the pad dimensions (L and B) have been replaced with dimensions for the two dimensional sector pad. The variation of W^* with film thickness ratio, H is shown in Figure 2-6 for $L/R = 2/3$

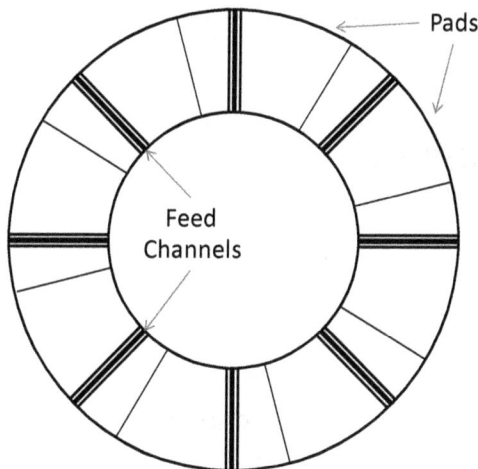

Figure 2-4   Tapered land thrust bearing with eight thrust pads and lubricant flow channels in between the pads.

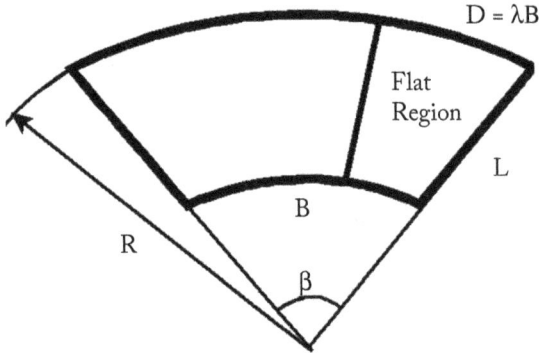

Figure 2-5 A 2-D tapered land thrust bearing pad with a pad extent of B and flat land section defined by extent D and width L.

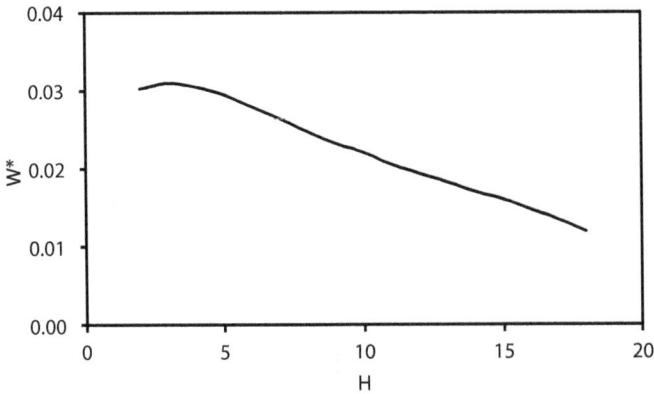

Figure 2-6 Non-dimensional load parameter versus film thickness ratio for a 2-D tapered land bearing with $L/R = 2/3$ and $\beta = 40$. Adapted from data in reference [6].

and sector angle $\beta = 40$, i.e., for an eight pad bearing. Note that the optimum load W^* is at $H = 3$. Note also that the normalized load is smaller in this case as compared to the simple one-dimensional bearings, due to side leakage. It can be shown that for a given viscosity the load capacity W/L increases with rotational speed ω and bearing radius R.

2.3 Journal bearings

Journal bearings used for load support in the radial direction operate with the same principle of the lubricant being forced into a converging gap. However, in this case the gap is developed during rotation of the shaft, as outlined below. In this bearing configuration, a cylindrical shaft, or journal, is supported in a circular cavity, or bush, which has a slightly larger diameter, Figure 2-7. The clearance (or the difference between the two radii) is usually less than 1% of the bearing radius. When the loaded bearing is at rest, the two centerlines line up in the vertical direction. As the loaded journal starts to rotate in presence of a viscous fluid a convergent wedge is formed in the direction of rotation. The fluid is drawn into the gap forcing the surfaces apart, Figure 2-7b, thus providing load support. Note that the center of the journal has moved towards the direction of rotation in Figure 2-7b. The exact solution for the journal bearing is too complex for presentation in this article. However, it suffices to say that the solution starts with the Reynolds equation and the pressure profile for a given bearing geometry is calculated. Special considerations are also given for the length of the bearing, side leakage, thermal effects, and others.

Although the formulations for journal bearings can be expressed in terms of a non-dimensional load parameter W^*, it is usually expressed in terms of the Sommerfeld No. S

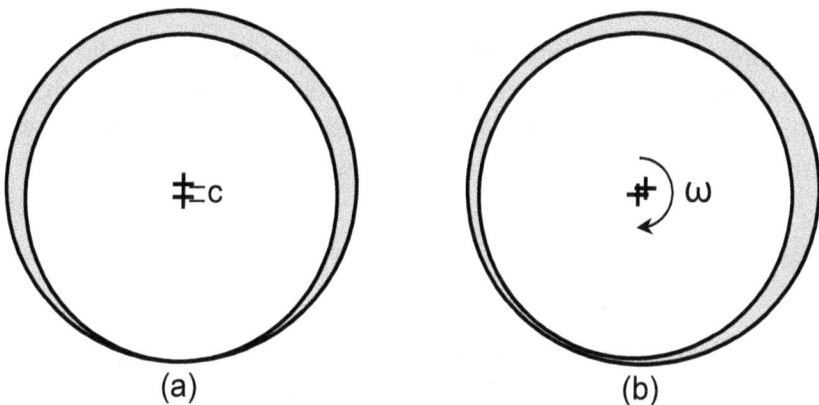

(a)　　　　　　　　　　　　(b)

Figure 2-7 Journal bearing loaded but no rotation in (a), and with rotation in (b). Note that the centers of the journal and bushing are lined up vertically in (a) but the bearing center is offset to the left due to rotation in (b). Note that the dimensions are not to scale; the minimum gap depends on viscosity and speed, and ranges from a few to several tens of micrometers.

$$S = \eta\omega\frac{LD}{W}\left(\frac{R}{c}\right)^2 \tag{2-7}$$

Where ω is the rotational speed of the journal, L, D and R are the length, diameter and radius of the bearing, respectively and c is the radial clearance, i.e., the difference between the radius of the journal and the bearing. For an infinitely long bearing, i.e., no side leakage,

$$\frac{1}{S} = \frac{6\pi\epsilon}{(1-\epsilon^2)^{1/2}(2+\epsilon^2)} \tag{2-8}$$

If eccentricity, or the distance between the centers of the journal and bearing, is designated as e, the eccentricity ratio ϵ can be defined as

$$\epsilon = \frac{e}{c} \tag{2-9}$$

Note that the minimum film thickness for a journal bearing can be defined as

$$h_{min} = c\,(1-\epsilon) \tag{2-10}$$

The effects of eccentricity ratio on Sommerfeld No. S, non-dimensional load parameter W^*, and attitude angle ψ between the load vector and the line joining the centers of the journal and bearing are shown in Figure 2-8. The load parameter is defined as

$$W^* = \frac{W/L}{\eta R\omega}\left(\frac{c}{R}\right)^2 \tag{2-11}$$

The load capacity (i.e., inverse of Sommerfeld No.) increases as the eccentricity ratio is increased. Also the attitude angle decreases, which means that the journal moves further up in the direction of rotation. Equations 3-13 provide guidelines for design of hydrodynamically lubricated thrust and journal bearings. An example for design of a blood lubricated thrust bearing is provided in Section 2.6.

2.4 Shear stress and hemolysis

Hemolysis refers to a medical condition in which the red blood cells are ruptured and hemoglobin is released into the blood plasma [7]. While

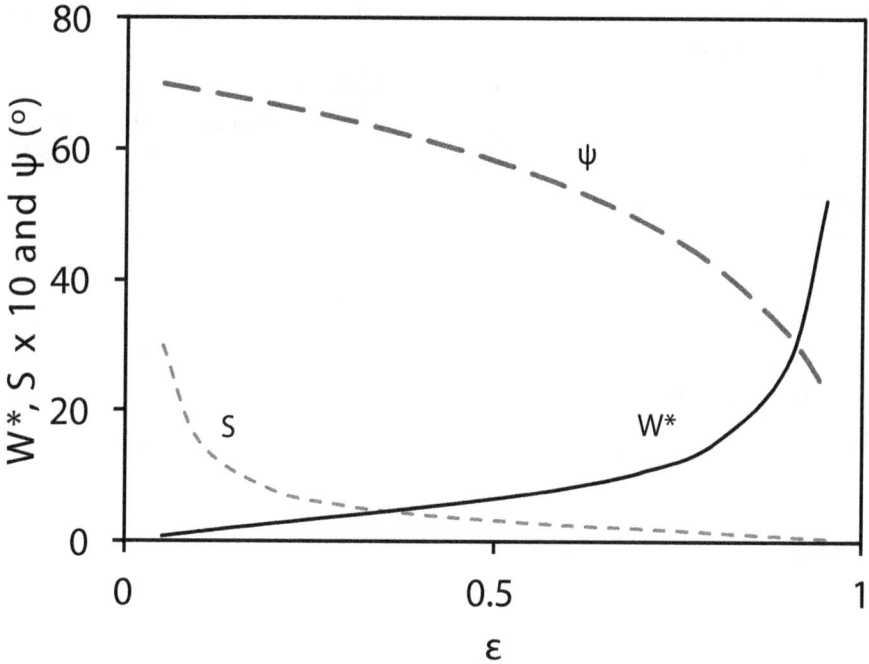

Figure 2-8 Non-dimensional load parameter W^*, Sommerfeld No. S, and angle ψ plotted versus eccentricity ratio ε for an infinitely long journal bearing. Data from reference [6].

there are many medical conditions, including genetic disorders that cause hemolysis, here our interest is in stress-driven cell rupture due to excessive shear, such as in mechanical bearings. Load carrying capacity of a hydrodynamically lubricated bearing is strongly influenced by the fluid film thickness, as described above. Since very small lubricant film thicknesses are usually required for load support, it is important to analyze the shear stresses that develop in the bearing gap so that high stresses that could cause blood trauma can be avoided.

According to Equation 1-2, shear stress in a bearing gap increases with viscosity and speed, and decreases with an increase in film thickness. This implies that shear stress in small bearing gaps could be quite high. This is an important consideration for bearing design, since large shear stresses in small bearing gaps give rise to higher temperatures and power loss, and in blood pumps could accentuate blood damage and hemolysis. Therefore, for a given fluid viscosity, the bearing gap or the fluid film thickness must be balanced to achieve the required load support and yet avoid high shear stresses.

Equation 1-2 has been derived for a cylinder rotating inside a journal with a constant gap. While it illustrates the basic relationship between shear stress, speed and film thickness, it needs to be modified for hydrodynamic bearing configurations. Considering again the tapered bearing in Figure 2-2a and define a non-dimensional tangential force [6] as

$$F^* = \frac{Fh_o}{B\eta UL} \tag{2-12}$$

It can be shown that F^* decreases as film thickness ratio H is increased.

$$F^* = 4\frac{\ln H}{H-1} - \frac{6}{H+1} \tag{2-13}$$

It then follows that the shear stress

$$\tau = \frac{F}{BL} = F^*\eta\frac{U}{h_o} \tag{2-14}$$

Note that the form of this equation is similar to the previous simple analysis (Equation 1-2), but the shear stress here is modified by value of F^*. The numeric value of non-dimensional tangential force F^* is equal to 0.745 at the optimum tapered bearing configuration, i.e., for $H = 2.3$.

The models and experimental results for stress driven hemolysis generally agree that the amount of blood damage depends on both the magnitude of shear stress and the time of exposure to shear, Table 2-1. The data listed in this table clearly indicate that a combination of exposure time and shear stress magnitude has to be considered for the determination of hemolysis. The data in the Table has been plotted in Figure 2-9, which shows that the threshold stress limit, below which no hemolysis occurs, is related to the exposure time. The hemolysis threshold limit increases as the exposure time is decreased. Although the empirical hemolysis model developed by Giersiepen et al. [8] and Wurzinger et al. [9], which is widely used, does consider both the exposure time and shear stress levels, it does not explicitly account for the damage threshold.

$$\frac{\Delta Hb}{Hb} = 3.62 \times 10^{-7} t^{0.785} \tau_{ave}^{2.416} \tag{2-15}$$

Table 2-1 Blood viscosity and damage stress threshold.

	Type of Exposure	Exposure Time (s)	Damage Threshold (Pa)	Reference
1	Rotating Viscometer	1200	60	Shapiro and Williams [10]
2	Concentric Cylinder Viscometer	9000	50 – 100	Sutera et al. [11]
3	Concentric Cylinder Viscometer	120	150	Leverett et al. [12]
4	Concentric Cylinder Viscometer	240	250	Sutera and Mehrjardi [13]
5	Concentric Cylinder Viscometer	120	300	Nevaril et al. [14]
6	Jet	$\sim 10^{-4}$	400	Sallam and Hwang [15]
7	Pulsating Gas Bubble	$\sim 10^{-3}$	450	Rooney [16]
8	Oscillating Wire	$\sim 10^{-3}$	560	Williams and Hughes [17]

Source: Adapted from Anderson et al. [18].

Here, ΔHb is the increase in the free hemoglobin in plasma, t is time of exposure to shear stress in seconds, and τ_{ave} is the average value of shear stress (in Pascal) during stress exposure.

For hemolysis analysis in blood lubricated bearings, this empirical hemolysis model should be extended to include the threshold value of shear stress below which no hemolysis occurs. Since the residence time in hydrodynamic bearings is expected to be in the milliseconds range, a threshold value of 200 Pa is assumed as the safe threshold value to be consistent with the data in Figure 2-9. Therefore, Equation 2-15 can be used when $\tau_{ave} > 200$ Pa; and for $\tau_{ave} < 200$ Pa

$$\frac{\Delta Hb}{Hb} = 0 \tag{2-16}$$

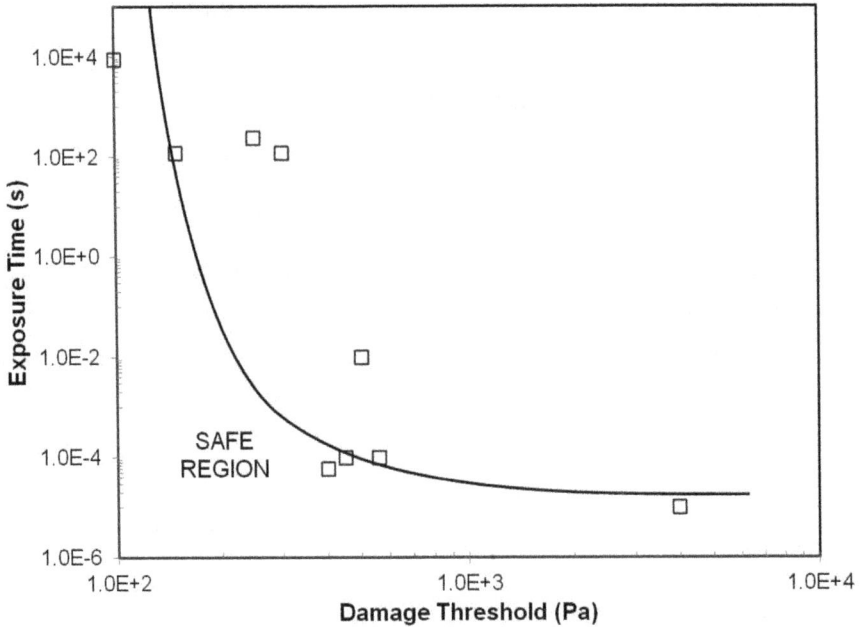

Figure 2-9   Shear stress damage threshold plotted as a function of exposure time based on data in Table 2-1 and reference [18].

A two-step engineering approach can be used for quantitative prediction of the rate of blood damage in hydrodynamic bearings. First, the Reynolds and continuity equations are used to determine flow rate and shear stress field in the shear driven fluid film formed by the blood, wherever Reynolds equation is convenient and valid. The fluid flow equations are also used on large gaps where hydrodynamic films are not formed to determine the remaining blood flow rate and corresponding shear stress field. Then, a set of boundary conditions and limiting parameters for the hemolysis equations are imposed. The values of τ_{ave} and t in the hemolysis model can be determined from the computed flow properties, for example for a particular thrust bearing configuration. The following section provides the basic steps used in the design and testing of a blood lubricated tapered-land thrust bearing for a rotary centrifugal LVAD with analysis for hemolysis potential. The design process starts with establishing the required load capacity, overall size envelope, and range of rotational speeds. Once an initial design is obtained, the bearing geometry is optimized to maximize the load capacity and minimize the potential for hemolysis.

2.5 Design and testing of a thrust bearing

The design and testing of the backup hydrodynamic thrust bearing in MiTiHeart® LVAD is used as an example. The cross-section of this LVAD is shown in Figure 2-10. The MiTiHeart® LVAD is a third generation, direct drive, centrifugal blood pump developed as destination therapy for adult heart failure patients [19–21]. This LVAD uses a hybrid passive/active magnetic bearing system with only one actively controlled axis (in the axial direction) to minimize the total bearing power draw and provide washing flow and low hemolysis (normalised index of hemolysis, NIH less than 0.002 mg/dL) [22]. The magnetic bearing system consists of a set of permanent magnet rings on both the rotor and stator, and magnetic coils on the stator. The passive forces between the rotor and stator magnets support the shaft in the radial direction and produce an axial bias flux. The axial force generated by

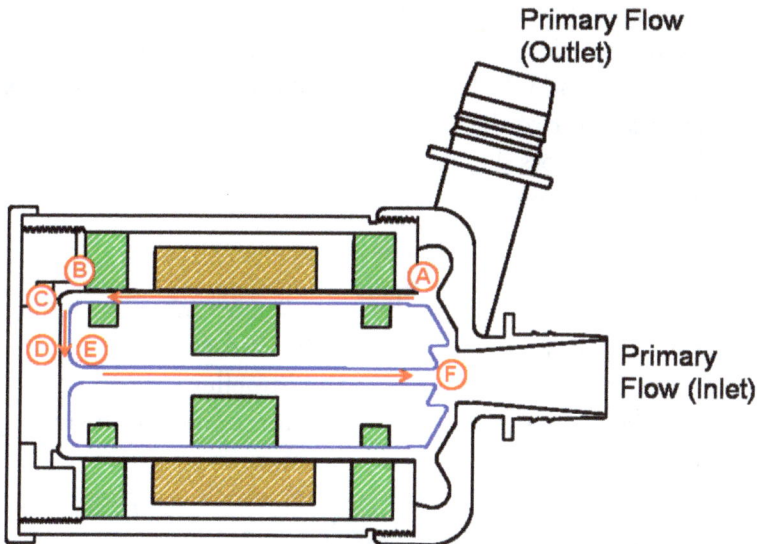

Figure 2-10 Secondary flow path in the blood pump prototype between rotor and stator (A-B), corner (B-C), thrust bearing (C-D), corner (D-E), and return flow (E-F). The motor stator is shown in brown and the magnets and coils for the motor and bearings are shown in green.

the electromagnets is actively controlled using a PID (proportional-integral-derivative) controller with zero-force balance to stabilize the rotor and minimize the power loss. In this LVAD design only one sensor is needed in the axial direction, as opposed to other active magnetic bearing designs [23] that use five active axes (one axial, two radial and two tilt) to provide complete control of the pump rotor during operation.

MiTiHeart® LVAD uses simple and direct flow paths for both main and secondary blood flows. The non-contact nature of the magnetic bearing allows for a fully washed secondary flow path to avoid stagnation points that might promote thrombi formation. The secondary blood flow path follows along the length of the rotor within the gap between the rotor and stator (A-B). The flow passes over the auxiliary hydrodynamic thrust bearing (C-D) and is forced to return to the impeller through a central cylindrical hole in the middle of the rotor (E-F) due to the differential pressure.

Clearances between the rotor and stator in the secondary flow path are designed to minimize hemolysis potential by reducing shear stress related activation of the coagulation processes [24]. Heat generation and hot spots are not significant issues, due to the low power levels and large surface areas available for heat dissipation. Cooling flow passes over the inner diameter of the motor and there are no rubbing contacts to produce local hot spots due to friction.

The rotor of the magnetically supported LVAD is subject to a number of axial forces:

1. Magnetic force generated by permanent magnets, which increases linearly with zero value at the mid-point,
2. Forces due to blood pressure at the impeller side and at the opposite side of the rotor; with the net force from both sides acting towards the impeller,
3. Dynamic forces due to rotor inertia, which are proportional to mass of the rotor and to the acceleration,
4. Dynamic forces due to viscous damping, most likely proportional to the instantaneous velocity with an unknown proportionality constant, and
5. Magnetic forces generated by active magnetic bearing, which are proportional to the magnetic bearing current with a proportionality constant.

Under normal operation of the LVAD, axial force balance of the system is fully ensured by the active magnetic bearing, which automatically adjusts the axial position of the rotor to such a location at which the resultant axial force from all the components is close to zero and the axial stability of the rotor is ensured. However, the backup hydrodynamic thrust bearing becomes essential if the rotor is pushed towards the back of the stator with a large axial force, for examples, in case of a severe shock or if the active magnetic bearing fails. The thrust bearing is located in the housing acting on the rear of the rotor, shown as segment "C-D" in Figure 2-10.

It was estimated that the thrust bearing, in this example, should be able to carry approximately 10 N to counter the mass of the rotor and the force of fluid entering into the LVAD. A tapered land thrust bearing (Figure 2-4) with an outside diameter of 4 to 5 cm was selected and the rotor speed of 3,000 rpm was assumed. The following nominal bearing parameters were used for analysis: R_i = 13 mm, R_o = 20 mm, A_P = 0.6 cm^2, β = 30°, eight thrust pads; where R_i and R_o are the bearing inner and outer radii, A_P is the effective pad area with width L and extent B.

Using Reynolds equation and the bearing analysis concepts described in the previous sections, the bearing pad geometry and film thickness were numerically estimated for the required load capacity and the boundary conditions of speed and geometry. Several bearing designs (different bearing extents, flat land dimensions, and ramp slopes) were evaluated. The first design was optimized for minimum levels of peak shear stress (designated as Bearing #1) and a second design was optimized for minimal levels of hemolysis (Bearing #3). Since minimizing the peak shear stress and minimizing the level of hemolysis lead the bearing design strategies in opposing directions, an intermediate design (Bearing #2) was also evaluated as a compromise between Bearing #1 and Bearing #3. Finally, a baseline design (Bearing #0) was considered with a linear ramp, while the other three designs had a slightly convex ramp.

An example of the bearing ramp slopes and flat land is shown in Figure 2-11. Note that the bearing pad extent B is in millimeters and the height h is in micrometers. The calculated pressure profile on one pad using the governing lubrication equations is shown in Figure 2-12. The aforementioned bearings were fabricated for testing. The fabricated

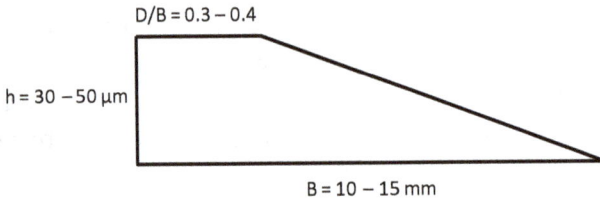

Figure 2-11 Typical tapered land thrust bearing configuration used for the design.

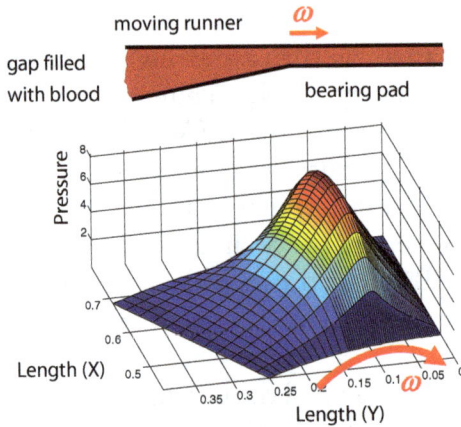

Figure 2-12 Hydrodynamic pressure buildup on bearing pad. Pressure intensity is shown in color from blue to red.

test bearings also included supply inlet ports to feed the lubricant near each ramp, Figure 2-13.

A thrust bearing tribometer (Figure 2-14) was used to experimentally verify the load capacity of the designed bearings. The thrust bearing housing was mounted on a frictionless rotary hydrostatic air table. The thrust runner was mounted to a variable-speed electric motor shaft. Prior to testing, the runner and the thrust bearing parallel alignment was verified using a dial indicator mounted to the thrust runner/ motor spindle assembly and contacting the thrust bearing manifold. The thrust runner was slowly rotated so that the dial indicator swept through 360° and indicated less than ±10 μm deviation at a 7.6 cm radius. Following alignment, lubricant film thickness (or bearing gap) calibration was completed by pressurizing the air table and adjusting

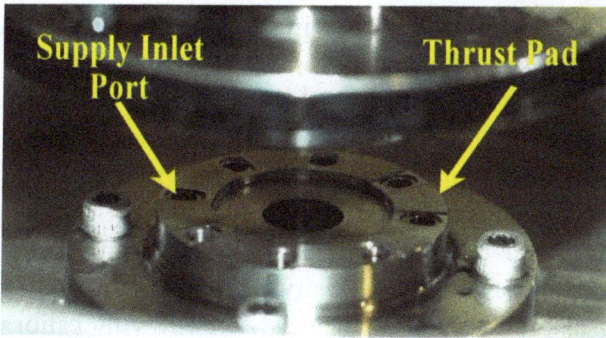

Figure 2-13 Prototype hydrodynamic thrust bearing for MiTiHeart® LVAD.

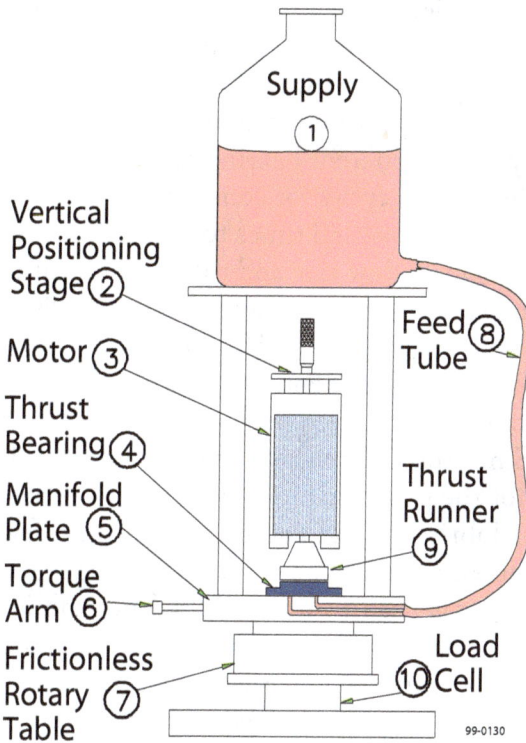

Figure 2-14 Schematic diagram of thrust bearing tribometer.

the vertical position until the first indication of contact was recorded by a load cell (Sensotec load cell, Honeywell, Morristown, NJ). The micrometer position was used to establish the zero film thickness point for all thrust bearing tests. The micrometer was used also to achieve the desired film thickness for bearing performance testing.

Bearing performance (i.e., load capacity and bearing torque) was assessed with a water-based lubricant, as a blood analog (a mixture of water and glycerol) having a viscosity of 3.5 cP, which is equivalent to the viscosity of blood at high shear rates. Following calibration of the system, the lubricant container mounted above the test section was filled and the bearing gap was set to a large value of 200 µm to 250 µm. Once the motor test speed (3,000 rpm) was established and lubricant flow was initiated, the bearing gap was slowly reduced to about 10 µm. During this loading cycle, the load capacity increased as the bearing gap or the lubricant film thickness was decreased. Once a small lubricant film thickness was achieved, the test was reversed by increasing the gap thickness. The load decreased during the unloading cycle. The loading and unloading curves did not always follow each other due to a small hysteresis in the vertical positioning actuation of the spindle. The load carrying capacity of the different bearing designs were, therefore, compared only for the loading cycles for consistency.

Each test was repeated several times to verify the repeatability of the results (i.e., bearing load, flow rate and torque). Repeat tests conducted with each pair indicated that the measured load capacity and film thickness values can vary by as much as 10–15% due to variations in room temperature, tribometer alignment, evaporation of water from the mixture, and uncertainties associated with measurement of the load or the gap thickness. Since the differences in the measured values were fairly small, the tests for the pairs used for comparisons were conducted with fresh batches of lubricants and completed within a few hours to decrease the experimental variations.

The tribometer was used to measure hydrodynamic characteristics of the four bearing designs. The torque or traction force between the rotating runner and hydrodynamic thrust bearing was measured with a strain gage; the axial load was measured with a load cell; and rotor speed was measured with an optical speed sensor.

Typical experimental results for 3,000 rpm are compared with theoretical predictions (solid lines) in Figure 2-15. Bearing #1 delivers a high

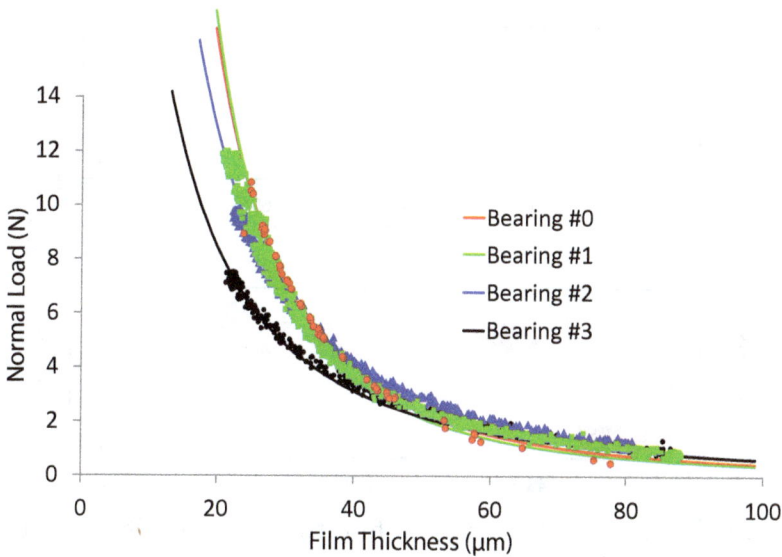

Figure 2-15 Bearing loads at 3,000 rpm for blood analog as a function of gap size. Theoretical predictions for the designs are shown by solid lines.

load of about 12 N at a gap of about 20 μm. The experiments showed that the measured load capacity agreed with theoretical predictions, albeit some variations due to the uncertainties in measurements. Design #1 was selected for further evaluation.

The next step in bearing performance evaluation is to determine the durability of the thrust bearing in constant load start/stop tests. The micrometer was disconnected from the system and replaced with a pulley and counter weight to vary the thrust load on the bearing. Static thrust loads were varied by adding or removing mass on the counter weight. Two loads of 4.5 and 8.9 N were used for these tests. Once the chosen load was applied to the bearing through the runner, the speed was increased from zero to 3,000 rpm and held constant until steady state was reached. The rotational speed was then ramped down to zero. Typical data for the start/stop durability tests are shown in Figure 2-16. The test begins with the bearing and the runner in intimate contact. As the speed is increased, the film thickness increases as hydrodynamic lubrication is established in approximately 3 s. When the speed is decreased to zero, film thickness decreases accordingly and the surfaces return to an intimate contact condition.

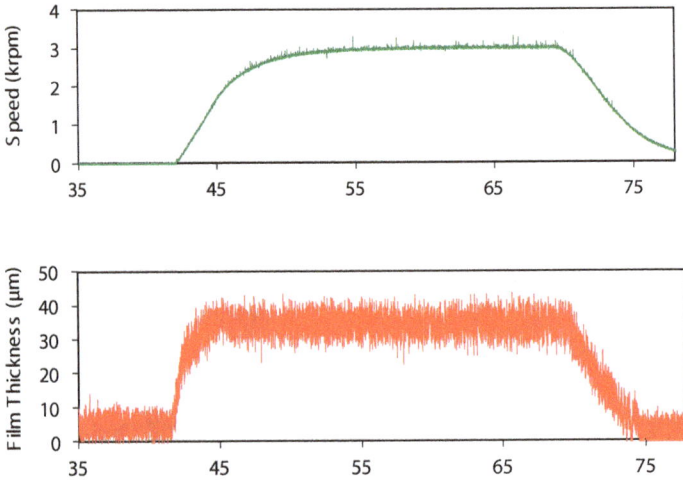

Figure 2-16 Typical speed and film thickness results from a single start/stop test on the hydrodynamic bearing.

The bearing surfaces examined after five test cycles at the lower load showed no sign of damage, except a few minor scratches. However, testing for five more cycles at 8.9 N resulted in a higher value of torque and surface damage in the form of a relatively wide scratch in the sliding direction. These results confirmed that while the designed thrust bearing would operate properly in the intended application, the use of several start/stop tests during implantation might cause permanent damage to the bearing.

Further tests were conducted to evaluate the bearing durability and validate the expected bearing function. In these tests, the bearing and runner were subjected to a series of impact (i.e., load-drop) tests designed to reproduce the same condition that could occur in the MiTiHeart® LVAD if magnetic bearing failure or a sudden axial shock were to occur. With only a slight load bias (< 0.9 N) toward the thrust bearing, the test runner was spun to 3,000 rpm. Due to the bias load, a large film thickness of 75 μm was initially achieved. When steady state was reached, a load of 8.9 N was quickly applied to the thrust bearing. These tests were repeated for five cycles. In order to make the load-drop test more severe, the load was then increased to 13.35 N, which was repeated five times.

Typical results shown in Figure 2-17 indicate that the dynamic load was larger than the load used in testing, and resulted in a sudden decrease in lubricant film thickness. The load oscillated and quickly stabilized in less

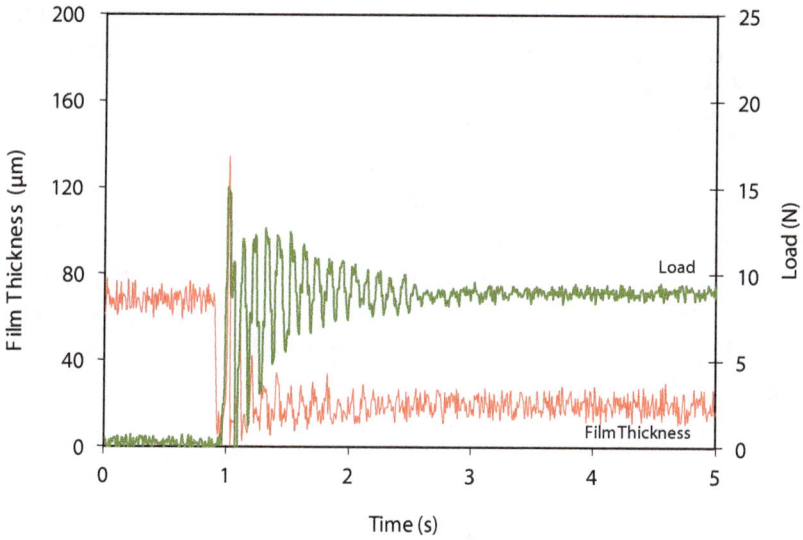

(a)

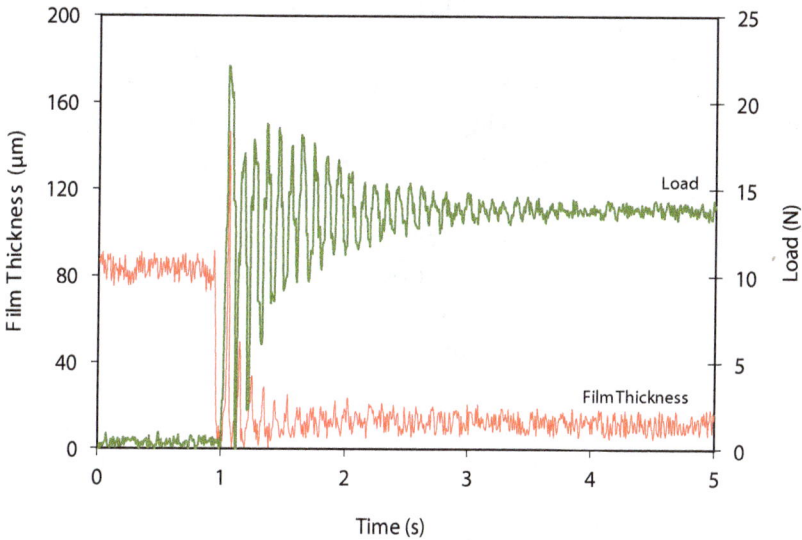

Figure 2-17 Change of lubricant film thickness and load in load-drop tests: (a) 8.9 N and (b) 13.35 N.

than 2 s. During this period, the lubricant film thickness almost reached zero for a short period of time. However, the thrust bearing quickly recovered and the lubricant film thickness increased to about 15 to 20 μm depending on the load. Note that the minimum film thickness, as stated in Section 1.2, should be larger than three times the roughness height, or at least 1 μm in this example. The titanium surfaces examined after these tests showed no sign of damage. However, when H-DLC (hydrogenated diamond like carbon) coating and/or heparin treated H-DLC were used on the bearing surfaces, the bearing durability in start/stop tests and in load-drop tests substantially improved, as no surface damage was observed following 50 start/stop tests and 10 load-drop tests [25]. The high hardness of H-DLC coating compared to that of the titanium alloy provides protection against wear and surface damage.

The next step is to model the amount of hemolysis generated by the chosen bearing design to ensure bearing performance based on hemolysis. Upon solving the Reynolds equation of lubrication for the bearing geometry and operating conditions, important parameters of the flow in the bearing were estimated. The computed parameters include pressure distribution, power consumption, levels of shear stress and total flow rate through the bearing. The leading edge of the pad (where blood enters) is divided into n sections of equal lengths, and blood flow rates Q_i entering the bearing are determined for each section $i = 1$ to n. A total of n streamlines are generated, starting in the middle of each section. It is assumed that what happens to blood along each streamline is representative of what happens to the blood flow rate Q_i along that streamline. An example streamline pattern (i.e., the paths followed by blood) consisting of $n = 12$ streamlines is shown in Figure 2-18. Along each streamline, the dependence of shear stress on time is determined, as well as the total residence time, i.e., time needed for blood to pass through the bearing along each streamline.

The flow rates and shear stress levels along the streamlines for Bearing #1 are shown in Figure 2-19. The stress along some of the flow lines exceeds the threshold value of 200 Pa by a substantial margin. However, the exposure time for these high stress conditions is less than 5 ms. The shear stress values along the streamlines are averaged, since the hemolysis model assumes constant shear stress values. This is simply done by integrating the time-dependant shear stress as the flow passes through the bearing along the streamlines, or

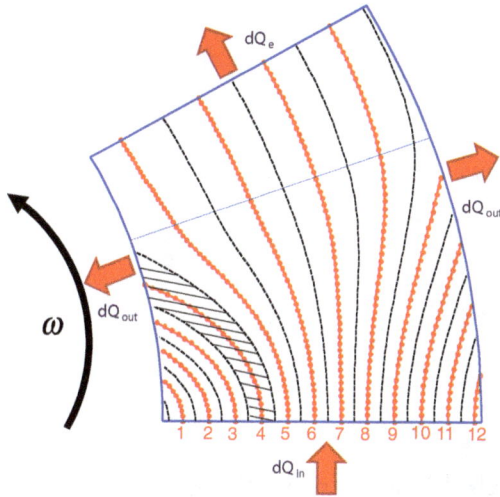

Figure 2-18 Flow pattern over one pad of the bearing.

$$[\tau_{ave}]^{2.416} = \frac{1}{t_{max}} \int_0^{t_{max}} [\tau(t)]^{2.416} dt \qquad (2\text{-}17)$$

The hemolysis equation is then used with the average shear stress and the residence time along each streamline. The hemolysis level (mg/s) for each streamline is determined by multiplying the flow rate along the streamline by the percentage of Hemoglobin in blood ($\approx$ 15 gm/dL) and by density of blood. To get the total hemolysis as the blood passes through the bearing pad, the hemolysis level is summed for streamlines $i = 1$ to n and then multiplied by the number of bearing pads.

The predicted levels of hemolysis for Bearing #1 are shown in Figure 2-20 as a function of bearing load. For the bearing size and conditions used in this example, the theoretical model predicts no hemolysis up to a load of 0.67 N during normal LVAD operation when the hydrodynamic thrust bearing is not engaged. Hemolysis level increases as the bearing load is increased. The normalized index of hemolysis for the fraction of blood that passes through the bearing can be calculated for a load of 8.9 N to be about 10 mg/dL (assuming a total flow of 100 L normally used for hemolysis testing. However, only a small fraction (less than 10%) of the blood passes through the bearing. Therefore, in this example the bearings contribute approximately 1 mg/dL to the

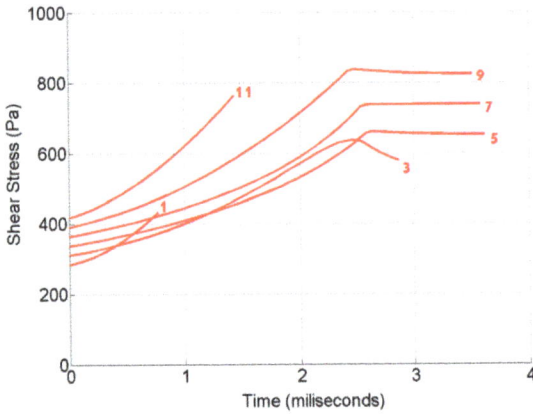

Figure 2-19 Shear stress along streamlines shown in Figure 2-18.

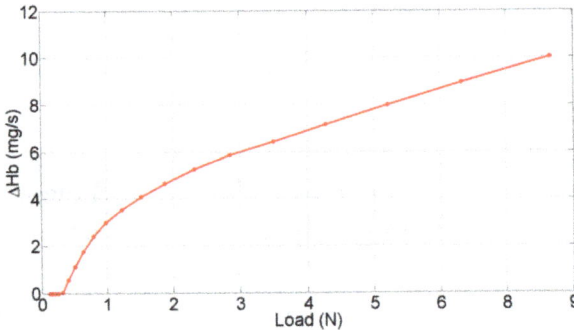

Figure 2-20 Predicted hemolysis levels for a particular thrust bearing design.

normalized index of hemolysis. Considering that a NIH value of 0.1 is acceptable for short term rotary blood pumps, the estimated contribution of the bearings when engaged should pose no problem for a short period of time that is needed for the patient to reach the hospital for corrective procedures. Since these calculations indicated that the estimated hemolysis potential of the selected bearing design is acceptable, bearing #1 was selected for implementation into the MiTiHeart® LVAD.

3. Lubrication of concentrated contacts

The types of bearings considered in the previous section possess "geometric conformity" between the two surfaces, e.g., two relatively flat surfaces in case of thrust bearings. Many machine elements, however, have curved surfaces, such as contacts between a cylinder or a sphere and a flat surface. In such contacts the pressure generated at the contact can be quite high and produce elastic (or reversible) deformation of the contacting bodies. For example, when an elastic spherical body is pressed against a rigid flat surface, the sphere will be deformed to form a flat contact between the two surfaces, as shown in Figure 3-1a. For a reverse case of a rigid sphere against an elastic flat surface, it is the flat surface that deforms to conform to the rigid sphere, Figure 3-1b. The dimensions of the deformed regions are highly exaggerated in the figure for visualization. In most cases however, elastic deformation takes place in both components. Such contacts between non-conformal surfaces

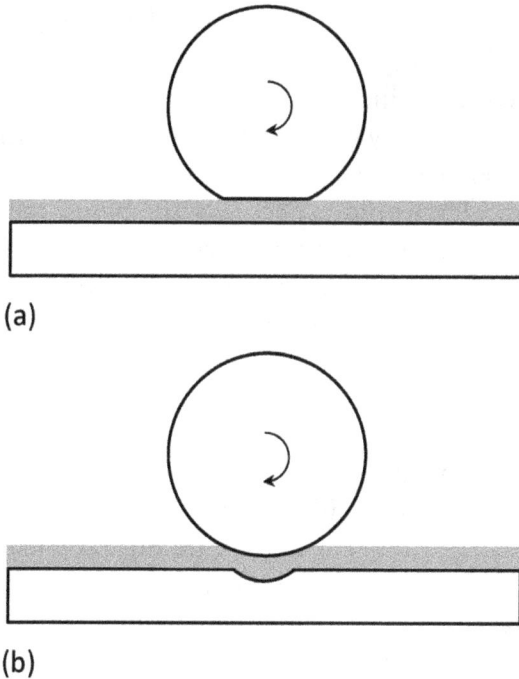

(a)

(b)

Figure 3-1 Elastohydrodynamic lubrication concept: (a) elastic deformation of the upper body, (b) elastic deformation of the lower body. Not shown to scale.

are often referred to as concentrated contacts, due to the large contact pressures on the order of GPa. The contacts in pivot bearings discussed in the Introduction (Section 1) fall in the category of concentrated contacts, and therefore this section is applicable to lubrication of such bearings.

3.1   Elastohydrodynamic lubrication

The Reynolds lubrication equation can be used to predict the load carrying capacity and lubricant film thickness in concentrated contacts. However, such calculations must consider the elastic deformation of the contacting surfaces. The formulation becomes rather complicated, as the local viscosity of the lubricant increase exponentially with pressure. The term "elastohydrodynamic lubrication" or EHL is used to describe the lubrication phenomena in such contacts. Typical examples include rolling element bearings and gears. The lubricant film thickness in such machine elements lubricated with mineral oils is generally on the order of 1 µm. Given that these surfaces are usually polished to a fine finish with a surface roughness better than 0.1 µm, the fluid film lubrication condition is established.

While the viscosity of lubricating oils can increase by several orders of magnitude [26], viscosity of water increases only slightly [27] at high pressures. However, viscosity of blood under extreme pressures has not been studied. One would expect that the blood cells would be destroyed under such high pressures. Furthermore, given the large size of red blood cells (6–8 µm diameter and 2 µm thickness), white blood cells (7–21 µm diameter) and platelets (2–3 µm diameter) it is unlikely that the cells would enter the small gap between the two concentrated contacts (less than 0.1 µm). Based on the effect of pressure on viscosity of water [27] one can surmise that viscosity of blood plasma may only increase slightly. In the absence of increased local viscosity in the contact, the fluid film thickness will be quite small and on the order surface roughness. Therefore, EHL conditions are not established for concentrated contacts lubricated with blood and the lubrication condition is expected to be in the boundary lubrication regime, where surfaces are in intimate contact with a molecular film in between them.

3.2   Boundary lubrication

It is instructive to first review the fundamentals of boundary lubrication before describing lubrication with blood in concentrated contacts, such as in pivot bearings. In boundary lubrication, the surfaces are in direct contact and only separated by a thin molecular film. Therefore, hydro-dynamic effects and rheological properties of the fluid are of little or no importance. The friction and wear properties of the contacting surfaces are primarily influenced by the physical and chemical interactions that take place between the solid surfaces and the molecular surface films. Surfaces are generally highly active and most species present in the en-vironment, in this case the lubricant, will be attracted to the surface. Molecules with polar groups are highly energetic and are strongly at-tracted to the surfaces, Figure 3-2. Such molecules include carboxylic acids (with –COOH groups) and alcohols (with –COH groups) or amines (with –NH2 groups) [28]. The adsorption process follows phy-sisorption (for example by hydrogen bonding, which is reversible) or chemisorptions (through irreversible bond breakage and chemical re-action). Various studies have shown that the coefficient of friction of

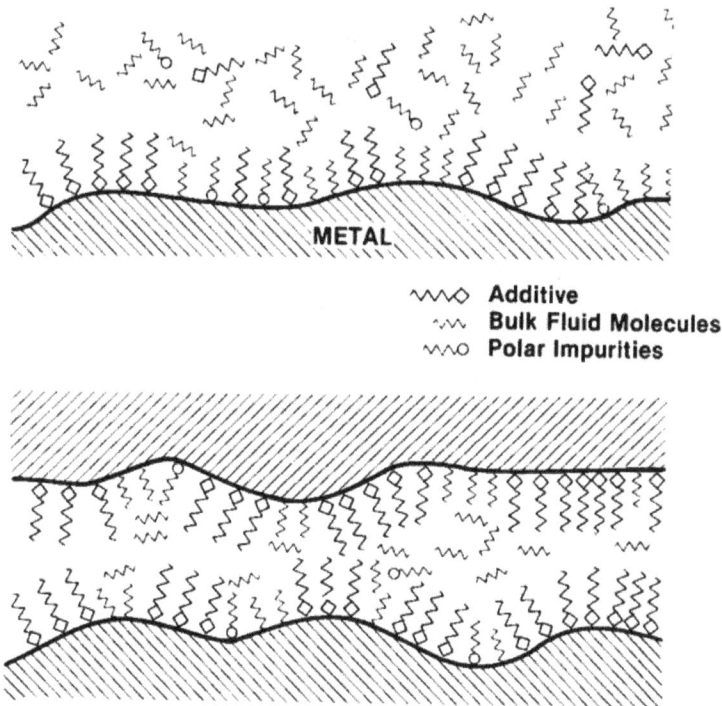

Figure 3-2   Adsorption of lubricant molecules on surfaces: (a) single surface and (b) two surface in sliding contact.

the carboxylic acids, alcohols and amines is related to the nature of the functional group and the length and structure of the molecule [29,30]. The carboxyl group has the highest adsorption strength followed by the hydroxyl and the amine groups.

The longer the hydrocarbon chain and the straighter, the higher is the adsorption strength due to intermolecular interactions [31]. While surface coverage of the polar molecules on surfaces increases with the concentration in the fluid, full surface coverage can be obtained at small concentrations, often less than 1%. The adsorbed molecules once achieved full surface coverage behave as a thin polymeric film protecting the sliding surfaces against friction and wear damage. It should be noted however, that the adsorption process is highly dynamic. Molecules are constantly adsorbed and desorbed from the surfaces with a residence time that depends on surface properties, molecular structure, temperature and pressure. Under adverse conditions of high loads or high temperatures, desorption rate would be higher and full surface coverage cannot be maintained [31]. When full surface coverage is obtained, with for example a high molecular weight carboxylic acid, the friction coefficient can be reduced from an unlubricated condition (usually ranging from 0.4 to 0.8 for most metal or ceramic combinations) to less than 0.1. Under similar sliding contacts, a non-polar hydrocarbon fluid would decrease friction to about 0.3 to 0.4. Control of friction has two primary benefits: lower contact heat generation and lower surface damage by wear. A reduction of friction from 0.4 to 0.1 reduces the wear rate by three orders of magnitude. Therefore, from the durability point of view for blood pumps, friction control is extremely important. Furthermore, it is crucial to control generation of wear particles from rubbing surfaces, since such particles can travel through the blood stream with catastrophic consequences to the patient.

Frictional studies have confirmed that the friction coefficient and wear rate of surfaces are lower in blood plasma compared to that in distilled water or buffered saline solution or under dry sliding conditions [32,33]. The lubricating property of blood plasma has been attributed to the presence of adsorbed proteins on surfaces. In vitro studies of materials used for artificial articulating joints have confirmed that addition of phospholipids to synovial fluid reduces the coefficient of friction [34]. Phospholipids are highly surface-active with polar functional end groups and long non-polar hydrocarbon chains, resembling commonly used industrial friction reducing additives, and form adsorbed surface layers. In addition to various proteins, amino acids and lactic acid, blood plasma also contains fatty acids with the carboxyl and hydroxyl groups. Although we are not aware of a thorough scientific study that has linked the lubricating property of bold plasma to its various constituents, one can clearly see how carboxyl, hydroxyl, and amine containing molecules would act as excellent boundary lubricants akin to those molecules studied as industrial lubricants.

3.3 Wear processes

When two surfaces are in intimate contact, irrespective of the contact geometry (conformal or counterformal), even with the presence of a molecularly thin boundary lubricant, surface damage and wear can result. It is instructive to review the fundamental mechanisms of wear in sliding contacts. Wear, by definition, is damage and/or removal of material from surfaces in relative motion. Surface damage or removal of material requires some form of energy, which could be in the form of mechanical, thermal or chemical [4]. Mechanical damage occurs through plastic or permanent deformation of the surface due to mechanical forces, i.e., normal contact load and friction force. Recall from the earlier discussion that the real area of contact is formed on the asperities, then deformation and fracture of the asperities or the material near the top surface of asperities constitutes mechanical wear [35], Figure 3-3. Wear damage is manifested in the form of displaced material rather than fracture, e.g., surface scratches. When surfaces are covered with oxides or other solid films, material removal takes place either inside the films or below the films depending on the contact conditions and the physical nature of surfaces. Mechanical forms of wear are highly sensitive to the contact

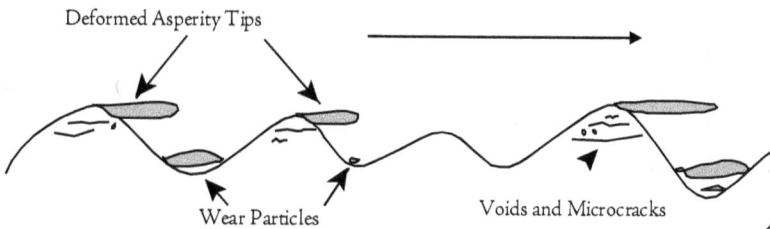

Figure 3-3 Deformation and fracture of surface asperities and generation of wear particles during sliding wear. Sliding direction of the counterface is from left to right.

stress and especially the friction coefficient. Generally, wear rate (measured as volume loss per unit sliding distance) is linearly proportional to the applied normal load [3]. However, there are exceptions to this rule, especially when chemical reactions take place at high loads or high speeds changing the nature and properties of the surfaces. Wear rate is usually related to the hardness of the material, since hardness is related to the capability of the material to deform plastically. In brittle materials such as ceramics, wear rate is related to both hardness and toughness of the material, where toughness is a measure of energy expended during fracture, or generation of wear particles [36]. As already discussed, reduction of friction through boundary lubrication has a pronounced effect on wear rate due to the reduction of tangential stresses at the contacting points [37]. It should be pointed out that wear is minimal for hydrodynamically lubricated bearings since no mechanical contact takes place during normal operation when the two surfaces are separated by a thick lubricant film (relative to the asperity heights). Wear and contact damage, however, occur when the two surfaces touch, for example during start or stop operation, or in case of shock loading.

Wear and surface damage also occur due to release of thermal or electrical energy at contacting surfaces. At high sliding speeds and when the friction coefficient is high, the elevated local temperature at the asperities (also referred to as flash temperature) can cause thermal damage, which is manifested in local softening or chemical reactions. This condition as arise when the boundary or hydrodynamic lubricant film is damage due to excessive loading. High speed contacts are also prone to the buildup and release of static charge and often generation of plasma, causing surface damage.

Given the potential for surface damage and wear when two surfaces are in n intimate contact, the most optimal condition is to keep the two surfaces apart, for example by hydrodynamic lubrication or magnetic bearings. Alternatively, if pivot bearings are used, it is crucial to design the contact geometry to maintain low stresses and to select hard wear resistant materials and or coatings.

4. Blood lubricated bearings in cardiac assist devices

Ventricular assist devices are divided into two types: paracorporeal and implantable. The paracorporeal devices reside outside the body with percutaneous blood flow lines. Most of these devices are based on centrifugal pumps. The implantable devices are segregated into three distinct design generations, delineated mostly by their bearing design. The first generation of mechanical circulatory assist devices was based on positive-displacement type pumps and avoided the need for blood contacting bearings. These devices are larger in volume, require greater input power and have more moving parts compared to their newer rotary counterparts [38,39]. The positive displacement pumps were the only option available for many years, in large part, due to the tremendous challenge of designing blood immersed bearings for rotary pumps. The rotary pumps are divided into two types: the second generation devices that use blood lubricated bearings, and the third generation devices that replaced the mechanical bearings with magnetic bearings. The rotary pumps are further divided into axial and radial pumps. Whereas the axial pumps generate high flow against low pressures, the radial or centrifugal pumps are capable of producing high pressures and low flows. In this section the types of bearings used in the different VAD designs are described. It is generally difficult to find accurate published information describing the bearings used in specific devices due to the confidentiality of such information.

4.1 Bearings in paracorporeal devices

Examples of paracorporeal pumps are listed in Table 4-1, which is mostly based on listing provided by Reul and Akdis [40]. These pumps used for cardiopulmonary bypass and for short term support use various types of bearings. The Medtronic Bio-Pump, Figure 4-1a, uses a sealed hydrodynamic journal bearing made from polycarbonate. The CardiacAssist TandemHeart also uses a sealed polycarbonate journal bearing, but the bearing is purged with a sterile lubricating/cooling solution. Since in these pumps the bearings do not come into contact with blood, the bearings do not contribute to blood trauma. The Terumo Capoix, Figure 4-1b, and the Sarnes Delphin use sealed ball bearings. However, these pumps require a seal to ensure that the lubricating/

Table 4-1 Paracorporeal pumps.

Device	Bearing type	Material
Bio-Pump	Sealed hydrodynamic journal	Polycarbonate journal bearing
TandemHeart	Hydrodynamic – purged/sealed	Polycarbonate journal bearing
Capiox	Sealed ball bearings	ND*
Sarnes Delphion	Sealed ball bearings	ND*
Gyro Pump	Blood immersed Pivot contact bearing	Alumina/UHMWPE
RotaFlow	Radial mag bearing Blood immersed Pivot bearing	Sapphire ball polyethylene
Impella	Ball bearing inside the motor	ND*

* Not Disclosed

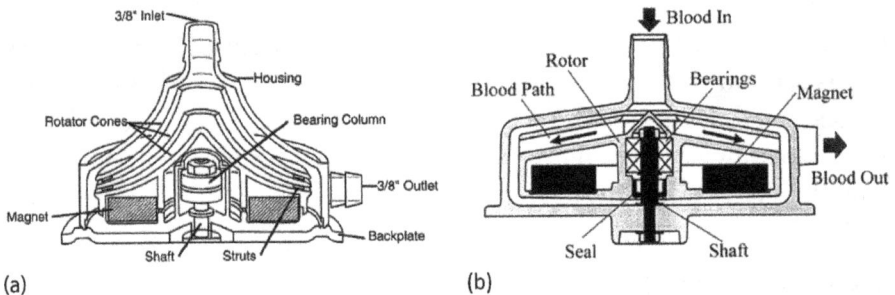

Figure 4-1 Cross section of (a) Medtronic Bio-Pump and (b) Terumo Capiox centrifugal pump [41,42].

cooling fluids do not enter the blood flow region of the pump. The flexible polymeric seals often produce heat generation and associated thrombus formation; therefore, these pumps are only used for short term support.

The blood immersed bearings found in some assist devices are based on contact bearings (i.e., pivot bearing), hydrodynamically lubricated journal or thrust bearings, and magnetic bearings. While the RotaFlow uses a combination of blood immersed pivot bearing and a radial magnetic bearing, the Gyro pump uses a blood-immersed, two-pivot contact bearing system consisting of high purity alumina ceramic balls rotating against ultrahigh molecular weight poly ethylene (UHMWPE) [43]. The ceramic balls are connected to a ceramic shaft. Systematic in vitro evaluations have shown that the ceramic/UHMWPE combination is superior to the ceramic/ceramic combination due to less wear, lower vibration and lower hemolysis [44–47]. The same studies estimated 5 to 10 years of bearing life depending on the application: cardiopulmonary bypass, left ventricular assist, or right ventricular assist. A variation of this design has been implemented for a small centrifugal pump for children and infants that uses a journal bearing configuration to support the impeller [48]. While the journal is made of polyethylene, the bearing shaft is made of titanium with a titanium ball end cap.

Impella, unlike the other radial pumps listed in the table, is an axial pump and uses rolling element bearings located inside the motor chamber and a polymeric lip seal. This pump is inserted percutaneously by minimal invasive surgical techniques through standard catheterization procedure. It is advanced into the ascending aorta, across the aortic valve, and into the left ventricle. A newer micro-axial version uses a combination of blood immersed sleeve bearings and a pivot contact bearing to provide radial and axial support [49]. Various material combinations were evaluated for durability and blood compatibility. Silicon nitride balls and shafts displayed a higher wear rate than zirconia. Several different polymeric materials, including UHMWPE, were evaluated for the sleeve bearing, but none performed well with respect to wear and mechanical integrity. The final selection of materials for the bearing system is not disclosed in the literature.

4.2 Bearings in the first generation VADs

While not employing blood immersed bearings, a number of first generation VADs did rely on mechanical bearings for their operation. Perhaps most widely known were the electrically driven Thoratec HeartMate XVE and the Novacor LVAS [50]. Unlike the pneumatically actuated positive-displacement devices, the electrically driven devices use electric motors (with imbedded bearings) and several linkages, drive pistons, or actuators that require mechanical bearings to act on the pusher plate to produce pulsating flow. These bearings were often the source of failure [51]. Examples of the drive systems and bearings are shown in Figure 4-2.

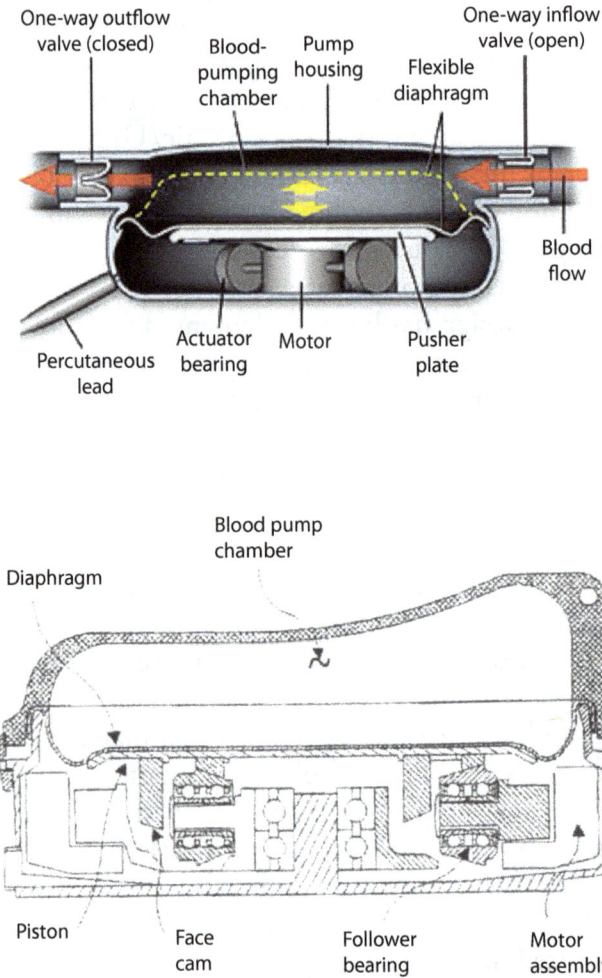

Figure 4-2 Typical construction of a pulsatile pump showing the motor and actuator that pulsate the flexible diaphragm, HeartMate [41,52,53].

4.2 Blood lubricated bearings in second generation VADs

The second generation assist devices, introduced in the 1990's [54–56], use different types of blood immersed contact bearing designs with reduced hemolytic and thrombolytic potential within the bearing.

These devices have since proven to be safe and reliable as demonstrated in recent long-term clinical successes [57–59]. Despite the numerous design enhancements afforded by the rotary blood pumps of the second generation, the blood immersed contact bearings in these devices are subject to inevitable wear degradation in long-term use.

The second generation axial flow VADs listed in Table 4-2 use a combination of blood immersed ceramic pivot and journal/sleeve bearings. While the Jarvik pump uses flat-ended contact bearings, the Thoratec HeartMate II and MicroMed DeBakey pumps rely on the ball and cup bearing design. These are shown in Figures 4-3–4-5. These bearings are usually placed on both ends of the rotating impeller, at the flow straighter and the flow diffuser. In the design of the blood-immersed bearing system for the Jarvik 2000 VAD, a sleeve bearing is used to provide radial support in addition to the use of pivot bearings that provide axial support. A pre-loaded satellite wire inside the rotor serves as the shaft with two silicon carbide sleeves serving as the journals [60]. Extensive in vitro testing has indicated potential for long term durability of this bearing system [61]. However, some design revisions were necessary for the smaller pediatric version of the Jarvik VAD due to bearing seizure and blood trauma experienced in animal testing [62].

To minimize the wear rate and ensure durability of the bearings for long term use in destination therapy hard ceramics such as silicon carbide or hard coatings such as TiC are usually used. An extensive search of the literature did not provide specific data on the wear rate or longevity of these bearings. Although the loads are relatively small and the rotational speed is very high (in the 7,000 to 15,000 rpm range),

Table 4-2 Contact bearings in second generation VADs.

Device	Bearing type	Material	References
Jarvik 2000 Flowmaker	Flat contact and sleeve	Diamond (or sapphire)	Jarvik [60], Marlinski et al. [61]
Debakey Heart	Ball and cup	Silicon Carbide	Noon and Loebe [63]
Heartmate II	Ball and cup	Ti-TiC Alumina	Maher et al. [64], Taylor et al. [65]

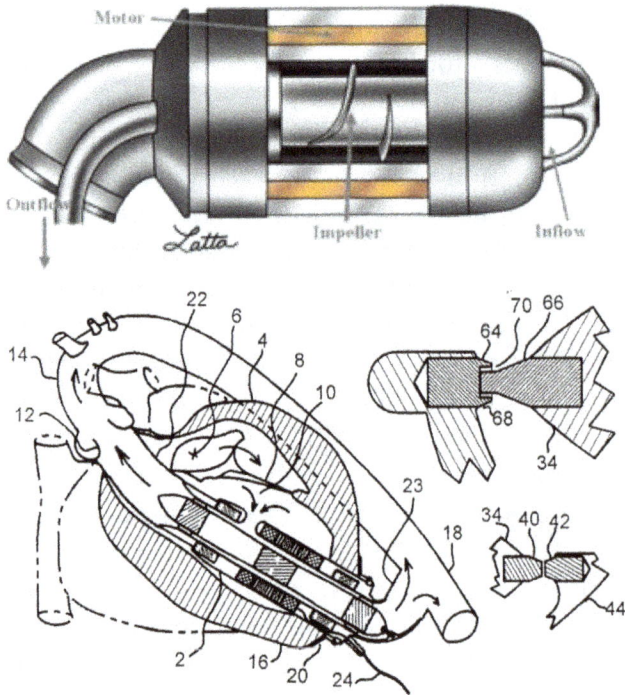

Figure 4-3 Cross sectional view of Jarvik 2000 and contact bearings (shown in the inset) [66,67].

the contact geometry of these pivot bearings is not conducive to the formation of a wedge that is needed for hydrodynamic lubrication. Therefore, these bearings operate in mixed lubrication regime or more likely in the boundary lubrication regime. However, given the high hardness of the ceramics or coatings used in these designs, the wear rates are probably low. In one study, housing vibrations due to bearing wear in an early version of HeartMate II has been reported [68]. More recent studies based on measurements of the wear on the explanted pumps after clinical trials have suggested that the pivot bearings in this VAD should provide an expected bearing life of at least five years [69]. While bearing failure and clot formation have been reported in a pediatric version of Jarvik Heart pump [62], the adult version of this device has been used in one patient for more than five years, indicating acceptable bearing life.

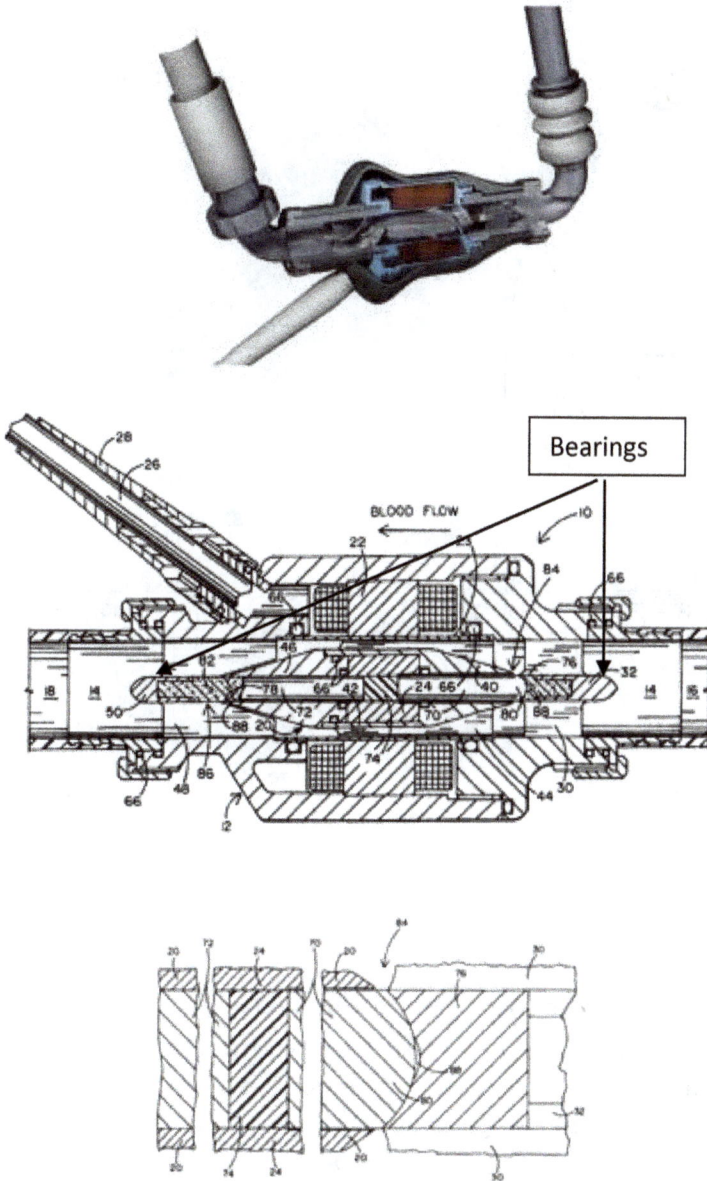

Figure 4-4 Ball & cup contact bearing used in Thoratec HeartMate II at both ends of the impeller [64,65].

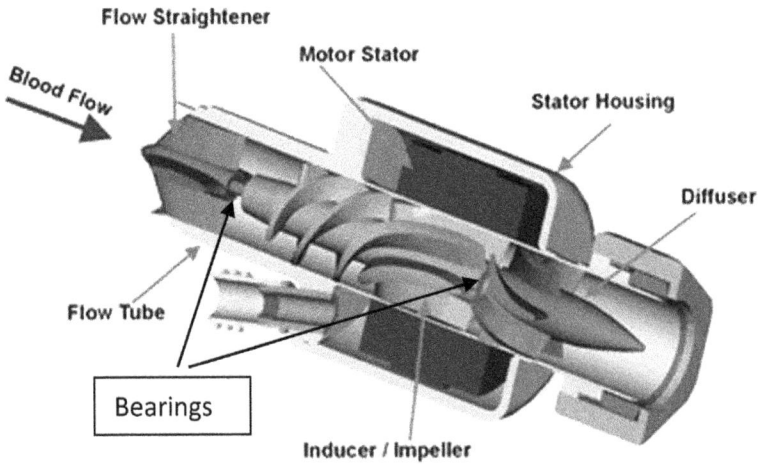

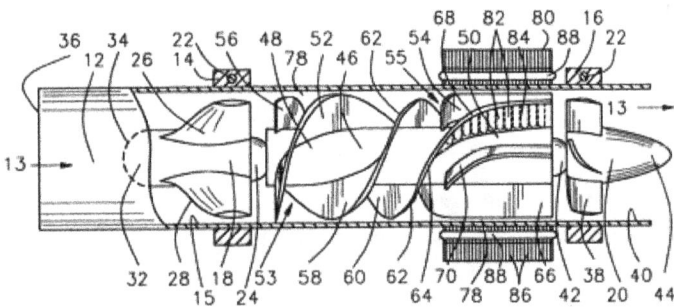

Figure 4-5   Locations for the ball and cup ceramic bearing in the MicroMed Debakey VAD, identified as numbers 24 and 42 [63,70].

4.3   Bearings in the third generation VADs

The third generation VADs is distinguished from second generation devices by the use of non-contacting bearings, typically magnetic or fluid lubricated hydrodynamic bearings (Table 4-3). As discussed earlier due to the lack of physical contact, these bearings are not subjected to wear during steady state use and offer the potential for limitless operation as destination therapy.

Although rolling element bearings relying on elastohydrodynamic lubrication are commonly used in most pumping applications, they are highly incompatible with the design requirements of an implantable blood pump. The high fluid pressures, high localized contact stresses

Table 4-3 Non-contact bearings used in third generation VADs.

Device	Radial bearings	Thrust bearings	Material	Reference
DuraHeart	Ball bearings in the motor	Passive magnetic	—	Hoshi et al. [71]
CorAide	Fluid lubricated - hydrodynamic	Passive magnetic	Coated titanium	Walowit et al. [72], Malanoski et al. [73]
VentrAssist	Fluid lubricated - hydrodynamic	Fluid lubricated - hydrodynamic	DLC coating	Waterson et al. [74], Qian and Bertram [75], Bertram et al. [76]
HVAD	Passive magnetic	Fluid lubricated - hydrodynamic	—	Wampler et al. [77]
MAVD	Passive magnetic	Fluid lubricated - hydrodynamic	Pt-Co rotor	Slaughter et al. [78]
MiTiHeart®	Passive magnetic	Primary – Active magnetic secondary - hydrodynamic	Titanium alloy	Jahanmir et al. [79], Jahanmir et al. [80]

and narrow passages can cause blood trauma. While a few specialized devices exist that use rolling element bearings for certain acute applications [40], no viable option has ever been presented for blood-immersed rolling element bearings for long-term support or destination therapy [81,82]. Rolling element bearings are, however, used external to the blood flow regions of the pump; an example is the motor bearings in Terumo DuraHeart [71], designed as an implantable VAD with magnetic bearings for destination therapy.

The CorAide VAD, Figure 4-6, uses a passive magnetic bearing in the axial direction and a hydrodynamic journal bearing at the interface between the rotating and stationary elements [83,84]. The journal bearing configuration has been designed to minimize shear stresses and increase the circumferential wash flow by creating a semi-elliptical bearing with the larger clearance (25 to 75 μm) located away from the loading point [72]. The nominal radial clearance for the journal bearing is about 75 micrometer [73]. While the main flow path is through the impeller housing, the secondary flow path follows the outside of the impeller and is returned to the main flow through a central axial hole, which also

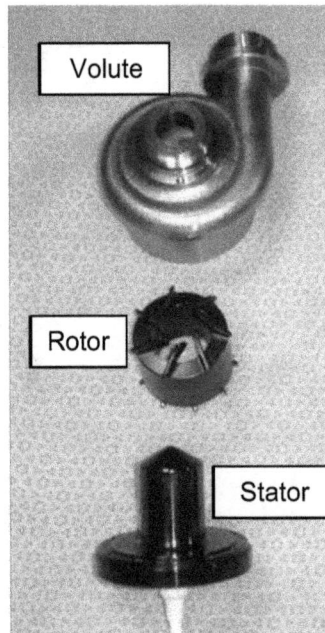

Figure 4-6   CorAide VAD components [83,84].

serves as the gap for the journal bearing. The rotor speed ranges from 1,800 to 3,200 rpm and a slightly modified version has been evaluated for right ventricular support [85].

The Ventrassist VAD uses blood lubricated hydrodynamic bearings to suspend the impeller, Figure 4-7. The front face of the housing is conical with a right angle apex, thus providing both radial and axial forces. The combined thrust and radial bearing in the form of a tapered wedge is integrated with each of the eight blades [74,86–88]. In addition, another 50 μm wedge is designed in the bottom of the impeller supporting thrust forces in that location as well. The gap between the blades and the upper housing ranges from 150 to 200 μm; whereas the gap between the impeller and the lower housing is 50 to 100 μm. The values for the bearing gaps are chosen to reduce blood trauma as the red blood cells with an average diameter of 8 μm pass through the bearing gaps. CFD analysis of the hydrodynamic bearings has provided confidence for the performance of the bearing system [75,76].

The HeartWare HVAD uses a passive radial magnetic bearing and a shrouded hydrodynamic thrust bearing [77]. The magnets are located within the impeller and the center post and are offset to keep the

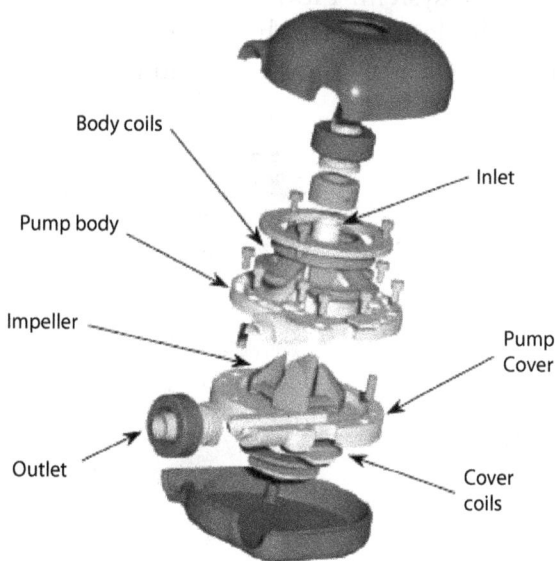

Figure 4-7 VentrAssit VAD components with the impeller in the middle [86–88].

impeller towards the front housing, Figure 4-8. Hydrodynamic lift is provided by the four tapered bearings on the impeller pushing the impeller away from the front housing. The primary flow path is through the inflow cannula and into four impeller flow channels after which blood is pumped through the outflow graft. The secondary flow starts under the impeller and goes upward through the annular gap between the impeller and center post and re-enters the main flow. The tertiary flow starts at the impeller slots and leads to hydrodynamic thrust bearings at the top of the impeller where blood re-enters the primary flow and exits the pump outlet [89]. The HVAD performance has been evaluated at speeds ranging from 2,400 to 4,200 rpm and the pump has been subjected to in vitro and in vivo animal studies prior to clinical evaluations [90]. The MVAD axial flow pump uses a radial passive magnetic bearing and a complex hydrodynamic thrust bearing design integrated with the impeller blades [78]. This design is shown in Figure 4-9. Having a smaller impeller compared to the HVAD, the pump speed ranges from 16,000 to 28,000 rpm.

The bearing design for the MiTiHeart LVAD was described in Section 2. This VAD uses a hybrid active/passive magnetic bearing as the primary bearing system. However, a secondary hydrodynamic bearing is used as a backup in case the magnetic bearing fails to operate properly. During normal pump operation the gap between the

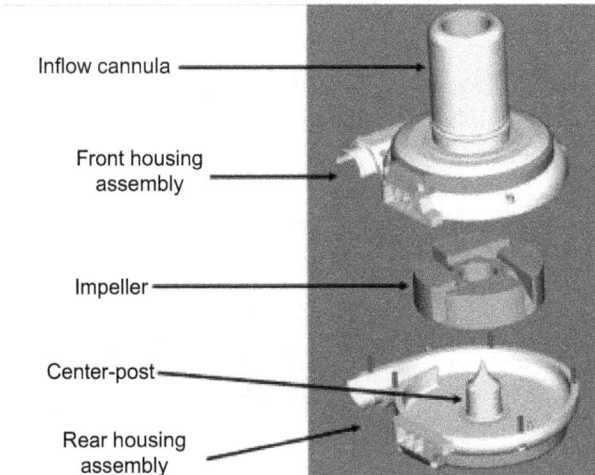

Figure 4-8   HeartWare HVAD components [77,89,90].

MOTOR STATOR

ROTOR

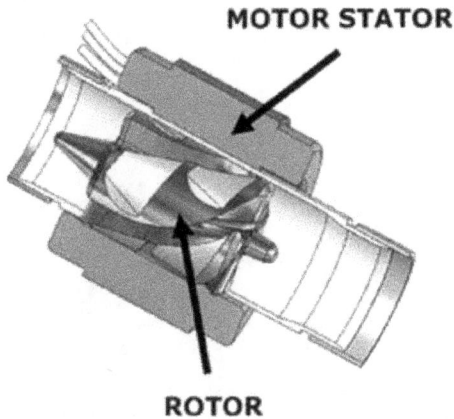

Figure 4-9   Blood lubricated hydrodynamic thrust bearings used in HeartWare MVAD [78].

bearing surfaces remains large and the hydrodynamic bearing is not activated. However, as the rotor is pushed toward the stator, the gap decreases and load support is enabled. The blood lubricated bearing, as described earlier, relies on a simple tapered land thrust bearing design. The MiTiHeart LVAD has been subjected to in vitro and in vivo animal studies to verify the performance and durability [79,80].

5. Concluding remarks

Mechanical circulatory assist devices have benefited from tremendous progress over the past decades since the first devices were introduced. Today, these devices, particularly those that have been approved by regulatory agencies for safety and effectiveness, are mostly safe and reliable, and provide a viable option for treating patients with serious heart related conditions. As in other mechanical systems, these devices require bearings to support the rotating and moving elements. This review provided a brief overview of different types of mechanical bearings and the principle design process. Some of the fundamental issues related to the potential damaging effects of wear and contact damage were discussed to highlight the importance of proper bearing design and selection of bearing materials for reliable and safe operation of the devices. The recent success in the design of these devices provides assurance that the future is bright and the assist devices will improve further and will incorporate new technologies as they become available for implementation.

Nomenclature

A_p = effective bearing pad area

B = bearing length, or bearing extent in the radial direction

c = journal bearing radial clearance

F = Friction force

F^* = non-dimensional tangential Force

h = lubricant film thickness

h_i = lubricant film thickness at bearing entry

h_o = lubricant film thickness at bearing exit

$\overline{h}$ = lubricant film thickness at location of maximum pressure

H = lubricant film thickness ratio, h_i/h_o

Hb = amount of free hemoglobin in plasma

L = bearing width

p = hydrodynamic pressure

R = radius

R_i = bearing inner radius

R_o = bearing outer radius

Q = fluid flow rate

S = Sommerfeld No.

U = velocity of a moving bearing surface

v_i = velocity of respective surfaces

W^* = non-dimensional load parameter

β = bearing sector angle

ΔHb = change in the free hemoglobin in plasma

ϵ = journal bearing eccentricity ratio

η = Lubricant viscosity

τ = shear stress

τ_{ave} = average value of shear stress

ψ = attitude angle between the load vector and the line joining the centers

ω = rotational speed

References

1. Neal, M. J., 1975, *Tribology Handbook*, Butterworth, London.
2. Blau, P. J., 1998, *Friction, Lubrication and Wear Technology*, ASM Handbook, Vol. 18, ASM International, Materials Park, OH.
3. Ludema, K. C., 1996, *Friction, Wear, Lubrication*, CRC Press, Boca Raton, FL.
4. Czichos, H., 1978, *Tribology*, Elsevier, Amsterdam.
5. Szeri, A. Z., 1998, *Fluid Film Lubrication*, Cambridge University Press, Cambridge.
6. Williams, J. A., 1994, *Engineering Tribology*, Oxford University Press, Oxford.
7. Maul, T. M., Kameneva, M. V., and Wearden, P. D., 2015. "Mechanical Blood Trauma in Circulatory-Assist Devices," *Biomedical & Nanomedical Technologies (B&NT): Concise Monographs Series, ASME Press New York.*
8. Giersiepen, M., Wurzinger, L. J., Opitz, R., and Reul, H., 1990. "Estimate of Shear Stress-related Blood Damage in Heart Valve Prostheses—in vitro Comparison of 25 Aortic Valves," *Artificial Organs*, **13**, pp. 300–306.
9. Wurzinger, L. J., Opitz, R., Blasberg, P., and Schmid-Schonbein, H., 1985, "Platelet and Coagulation Parameters Following Millisecond Exposure to Laminar Shear Stress," *Thromb Haemost*, **54**, pp. 381–6.
10. Shapiro, S. I., and Williams, M. C., 1970, "Hemolysis in Simple Shear Flows," *AIChE J.*, **16**, pp. 575–580.
11. Sutera, S. P., Croce, P. A., and Mehrjardi, M., 1972, "Hemolysis and Subhemolytic Alterations of Human RBC Induced by Turbulent Shear Flow," *Trans. ASAIO*, **18**, pp. 335–341.
12. Leverett, L. B., Hellums, J. D., Alfrey, C. P., and Lynch, E. C., 1972, "Red Blood Cell Damage by Shear Stress," *Biophys. J.*, **12**, pp. 257–272.
13. Sutera, S. P., and Mehrjardi, M. H., 1975, "Deformation and Fragmentation of Human Red Blood Cells in Turbulent Shear Flow," *Biophys. J.*, **5**, pp. 1–10.
14. Nevaril, C. G., Hellums, J. D., Alfrey, C. P., and Lynch, E. C., 1969, "Physical Effects in Red Blood Cell Trauma," *AIChE J*, **15**, pp. 707–711.

15. Sallam, A. M., and Hwang, H. C., 1984, "Human Red Blood Cell: Hemolysis in a Turbulent Shear Flow: Contribution of Reynolds Shear Stresses," *Biorheology*, **21**, pp. 783–797.

16. Rooney, J. A., 1970, "Hemolysis Near an Ultrasonically Pulsating Gas Bubble," *Science*, **169**, pp. 869–871.

17. Williams, A. R., Hughes, D. E., and Nyborg, W. L., 1970, "Hemolysis Near a Transversely Oscillating Wire," *Science*, **169**, pp. 871–873.

18. Anderson, J. B., Wood, H. G., Allaire, P. E., McDaniel, J. C., Olsen, D. B., and Bearnson, G., 2000, "Numerical Studies of Blood Shear and Washing in a Continuous Flow Ventricular Assist Device," *ASAIO Journal*, **46**, pp. 486–487.

19. Chen, H. M., 2001, "Pump Having Magnetic Bearing for Pumping Blood and the Like," US Patent No. 6,201,329.

20. Locke, D. H., 2004, "Combination Magnetic Radial and Thrust Bearing," US Patent No. 6,717,311.

21. Locke, D. H., Swanson, E. S., Walton, J. F., Willis, J. P., and Heshmat, H., 2003, "Testing of a Centrifugal Blood Pump with a High Efficiency Hybrid Magnetic Bearing," *ASAIO Journal*, **49**(6):737–43.

22. Ren, Z., Jahanmir, S., Heshmat, H., Hunsberger, A. Z., and Walton, J. F., 2009, "Design Analysis and Performance Assessment of Hybrid Magnetic Bearings for a Rotary Centrifugal Blood Pump," *ASAIO Journal*, **55**, pp. 340–347.

23. Bearnson, G. B., 1998, "Implantable Centrifugal Pump with Hybrid Magnetic Bearings," *ASAIO Journal*, **44**, pp. M733–736.

24. Hryniewicz, P., Willis, J. P., Jahanmir, S., and Heshmat, H., 2003, "Quantification of Blood Hemolysis Due to Mechanical Shearing," *ASAIO Journal*, **49**, pp. 217.

25. Jahanmir, S., Hunsberger, A. Z., and Heshmat, H., 2011, "Load Capacity and Durability of H-DLC Coated Hydrodynamic Thrust Bearings," *J. Tribology*, **133**(3), pp. 031301.

26. Booser, E. R. (Ed.), 1983, *Handbook of Lubrication*, CRC Press, Boca Raton, FL.

27. Stanley, E. M., and Batten, R. C., 1969, "Viscosity of Water at High Pressures and Moderate Temperatures," *J. Phy. Chem.*, **73**, pp. 1187–1191.

28. Beltzer, M., and Jahanmir, S., 1987, "The Role of Dispersion Interactions Between Hydrocarbon Chains in Boundary Lubrication," *ASLE Trans.*, **30**, pp. 47–54.

29. Jahanmir, S., and Beltzer, M., 1986, "An Adsorption Model for Friction in Boundary Lubrication," *ASLE Trans.*, **29**, pp. 423–430.

30. Jahanmir, S., and Beltzer, M., 1986, "The Effect of Additive Molecular Structure on Friction Coefficient," *J. of Tribology*, **108**, pp. 109–116.

31. Jahanmir, S., 1985, "Chain Length Effects in Boundary Lubrication," *Wear*, **102**, pp. 331–349.

32. Triolo, P. M., and Andrade, J. D., 1983, "Surface Modification and Characterization of Some Commonly Used Catheter Materials: II Friction Characterization," *J. Biomedical Materials Res.*, **17**, pp. 140–165.

33. Dangsheng, X., and Jin, Z. M., 2004, "Tribological Properties of Ion Implanted UHMWPE Against Si_3N_4 Under Different Lubrication Conditions," *Surface and Coatings Technology*, **182**, pp. 149–155.

34. Ozturk, H. E., Stoffel, K. K., Jones, C. F., and Stachowiak, G. W., 2002, "The Effect of Surface Active Phospholipids on the Lubrication of Osteoarthritic Sheep Knee Joint Friction," *Tribology Letters*, **16**, pp. 283–289.

35. Jahanmir, S., 1986, "On Mechanics and Mechanisms of Laminar Wear Particle Formation," *Advances in Mechanics and Physics of Surfaces*, Vol. III, R. L. Latanision and T. E. Fischer (Eds.) Harwood Press, New York, NY, pp. 261–332.

36. Jahanmir, S., 1994, *Friction and Wear of Ceramics*, Marcel Dekker, New York.

37. Jahanmir, S., 1985, "The Relationship of Friction Coefficient to Wear," *Wear*, **103**, pp. 233–252.

38. DeBakey, M. E., Liotta, D., and Hall, C. W, 1966, "Left Heart Bypass Using an Implantable Blood Pump," *Mechanical Devices to Assist the Failing Heart*, Proceedings of a Conference Sponsored by the Committee on Trauma, Sept 9–10, 1964, Washington DC, National Academy of Sciences-National Research Council, p. 223.

39. Giridharan, G. A., Lee, T. J., Ising, M., Sobieski, M. A., Koenig, S. C., Gray, L. A., and Slaughter, M. S., 2012, "Miniaturization of Mechanical Circulatory Support Systems," *Artificial Organs*, **36**(8), pp. 731–758.

40. Reul, H. M., and Akdis, M., 2000, "Blood Pumps for Circulatory Support," *Perfusion*, **15**, pp. 295–311.

41. Nose, Y., and Motomura, T., 2003, Cardiac Prosthesis—Artificial Heart and Assist Circulation. Volume III, 4th Edition, ICMT Press, Houston, TX.

42. Tayama, E., Raskin, S. A., and Nose, Y., 2000, "Blood Pumps," In *Cardiopulmonary Bypass: Principles and Practice*, 2nd edition, Chapter 3, Gravlee, G. P., Davis, R. F., Kurusz, M., and Utley, J. R. (eds), 2000 , Lippincott Williams & Wilkins, Philadelphia, PA.

43. Muramatsu, K., Masuoka, T., and Fujisawa, A., 2001, "In Vitro Evaluation of the Heparin-Coated Gyro C1E3 Blood Pump," *Artificial Organs*, **25**, pp. 585–590.

44. Nakazawa, T., Makinouchi, K., Ohara, Y., Ohtsubo, S., Kawahito, K., Tasai, K., Shimono, T., Benkowski, R., Damm, G., Takami, Y., Glueck, J., Noon, G. P., and Nosé, Y., 1996,"Development of a Pivot Bearing Supported Sealless Centrifugal Pump for Ventricular Assist," *Artificial Organs*, **20**(6), pp. 485–90.

45. Makinouchi, K., Nakazawa, T., Takami, Y., Takatani, S., and Nosé, Y., 1996,"Evaluation of the Wear of the Pivot Bearing in the Gyro C1E3 Pump. *Artificial Organs*, **20**(6), pp. 523–8.

46. Takami, Y., Nakazawa, T., Makinouchi, K., Benkowski, R., Glueck, J., and Nosé, Y., 1997, "Material of the Double Pivot Bearing System in the Gyro C1E3 Centrifugal Pump," *Artificial Organs*, **21**(2), pp. 143–7.

47. Takami, Y., Nakazawa, T., Makinouchi, K., Glueck, J., and Nosé, Y., 1997,"Biocompatibility of Alumina Ceramic and Polyethylene as Materials for Pivot Bearings of a Centrifugal Blood Pump," *J. Biomed. Mater. Res.*, **36**(3), pp. 381–6.

48. Takatani, S., Hoshi, H., Tajima, K., Ohuchi, K., Nakamura, M., Asama, J., Shimshi, T., and Yoshikawa, M., 2005, "Feasibility of a Miniature Centrifugal Rotary Blood Pump for Low-Flow Circulation in Children and Infants," *ASAIO Journal*, **51**(5), pp. 557–62.

49. Mahmood, A. K., Kerkhoffs, W., Schumacher, O., and Reul, H., 2003,"Investigation of Materials for Blood-Immersed Bearings in a Microaxial Blood Pump," *Artificial Organs*, **27**(2), pp. 169–73.

50. Goldstein, D. J., and Oz, M. C., 2000, *Cardiac Assist Devices*, Futura Publishing Company, Armonk, NY.

51. Patel, S. M., Throckmorton, A. L., Untaroiu, A., Allaire, P. E., Wood, H. G., and Olson, B. O., 2005, "The Status of Failure and Reliability Testing of Artificial Blood Pumps," *ASAIO Journal*, **51**, pp. 440–451.

52. Wilhelm, M. J., Ruschitzka, F., and Falk V., 2013, "Destination Therapy—Time for a Paradigm Change in Heart Failure Therapy," *Swiss Med. Wkly.*, **143**, 13729.

53. Slaughter, M. S., Rogers, J. G., Milano, C. A., Russell, S. D., Conte, J. V., Feldman, D., Sun, B., Tatooles, A. J., Delgado, R. M., Long, J. W., Wozniak, T. C., Ghumman, W., Farrar, D. J., and Frazier, O. H., 2009, "Advanced Heart Failure Treated with Continuous-Flow Left Ventricular Assist Device," *N. Engl. J. Med.*, **361**(23), pp. 2241–51.

54. Griffith, B. P., Kormos, R. L., Borovetz, H. S., Litwak, K., Antaki, J. F., Poirier, V. L., and Butler, K. C., 2001, "HeartMate II Left Ventricular Assist System: From Concept to First Clinical Use," *Ann Thorac. Surg.*, **71**, pp. 116–120.

55. DeBakey, M. E., 1999, "A Miniature Implantable Ventricular Assist Device," *Ann. Thorac. Surg.*, **68**, pp. 637–640.

56. Frazier, O. H., Myers, T. J., Westaby, S., and Gregoric, I. D., 2004, "Clinical Experience with an Implantable, Intracardiac, Continuous Flow Circulatory Support Device: Physiologic Implications and Their Relationship to Patient Selection," *Ann. Thorac. Surg.*, **77**, pp. 133–42.

57. Siegenthaler, M. P., Frazier, O. H., Beyerdorf, F., Martin, J., Laks H., Elefteriades, J., Khaghani, A., Kjellman, U., Pepper, J., Jarvik, R., and Westaby, S., 2006, "Mechanical Reliability of the Jarvik 2000 Heart," *Ann. Thorac. Surg.*, **81**(5), pp. 1752–8.

58. Park, S. J., Milano, C. A., Tatooles, A. J., Rogers, J. G., Adamson, R. M., Steidley, D. E., Ewald, G. A., Sundareswaran, K. S., Farrar, D. J., and Slaughter, M. S., 2012, "Outcomes in Advanced Heart Failure Patients with Left Ventricular Assist Devices for Destination Therapy," *Circ. Heart Fail.*, **5**(2), pp. 241–248.

59. Miller, L. W., Pagani, F. D., Russell, S. D., John, R., Boyle, A. J., Aaronson, K. D., Conte, J. V., Naka, Y., Mancini, D., Delgado, R. M., MacGillivray, T. E., Farrar, D. J., and Frazier, O. H., 2007, "Use of a Continuous-Flow Device in Patients Awaiting Heart Transplant," *N. Engl. J. Med.*, **357**, pp. 885–96.

60. Jarvik, R. K., 1995, "System Considerations Favoring Rotary Artificial Hearts with Blood-Immersed Bearings," *Artificial Organs*, **19**(7), pp. 565–70.

61. Marlinski, E., Jacobs, G., Deirmengian, C., and Jarvik, R., 1998, "Durability Testing of Components for the Jarvik 2000 Completely Implantable Axial Flow Left Ventricular Assist Device," *ASAIO Journal*, **44**(5), pp. M741–4.

62. Kilic, A., Nolan, T. D., Li, T., Yankey, G. K., Prastein, D. J., Cheng, G., Jarvik, R., Wu, Z. J., and Griffith, B. P., 2007, "Early in vivo Experience with the Pediatric Jarvik 2000 Heart," *ASAIO Journal*, **53**(3), pp. 374–8.

63. Noon, G. P., and Loebe, M., 2010, "Current Status of the MicroMed Debakey Noon Ventricular Assist Device," *Texas Heart Inst Journal*, 37, pp. 652–653.

64. Maher, T. R., Taylor, L. P., le Blanc, P. W. J. C., and Butler, K. C., 1998, "An Implantable Electric Axial-Flow Blood Pump with Blood Cooled Bearing," US Patent No. 5,707,218.

65. Taylor, L. P., le Blanc, P. W. J. C., Butler, K. C., and Maher, T. R., 1995, "Implantable Electric Axial-Flow Blood Pump," US Patent No. 5,588,812.

66. Anonymous, Texas Heart Institute, Department of Scientific Publications, http://www.texasheart.org/AboutUs/Depart/scipub.cfm, accessed August 2014.

67. Jarvik, R., 1994, "Artificial Hearts with Permanent Magnet Bearings," US Patent No. 5507629.

68. Butler, K., Dow, J., Litwak, P., Kormos, R., and Brovetz, H., 1999, "Development of Nimbus/University of Pittsburg Innovative Ventricular Assist System," *Ann. Thorac. Surg.*, **68**, pp. 790–794.

69. Butler, K. C., and Farrar, D. J., 2006, "No Bearing Wear Detected in Explanted Clinical HeartMate II LVADS," *ASAIO Journal*, 52, p. 33A.

70. Aber, G. S., 2001, "Method for Providing a Jewel Bearing for Supporting a Pump Rotor Shaft," US Patent No. 6,254,359.

71. Hoshi, H., Shinshi, T., and Takatani, S., 2006, "Third Generation Blood Pumps with Mechanical Non-Contact Magnetic Bearing," *Artificial Organs*, **30**(5), pp. 324–339.

72. Walowit, J. D., Malanoski, S. B., Horvath, D., Golding, L. R., and Smith, W. A., 1997, "The Analysis, Design and Testing of a Blood

Lubricated Hydrodynamic Journal Bearing," *ASAIO Journal*, **43**, pp. M556–M559.

73. Malanoski, S. B., Belawski, H., Horvath, D., Smith, W. A., and Golding, L. R., 1998, "Stable Blood Lubricated Hydrodynamic Journal Bearing with Magnetic Loading," *ASAIO Journal*, **44**(5), pp. M737–40.

74. Watterson, P. A., Woodard, J. C., Ramsden, V. S., and Reizes, J. A., 2000, "VentrAssist Hydrodynamically Suspended, Open, Centrifugal Blood Pump," *Artificial Organs*, **24**(6), pp. 475–7.

75. Qian, Y., and Bertram, C. D., 2000, "Computational Fluid Dynamics Analysis of Hydrodynamic Bearings of the VentrAssist Rotary Blood Pump," *Artificial Organs*, **24**(6), pp. 488–91.

76. Bertram, C. D., Qian, Y., and Reizes, J. A., 2001, "Computational Fluid Dynamics Performance Prediction for the Hydrodynamic Bearings of the VentrAssist Rotary Blood Pump," *Artificial Organs*, **25**(5), pp. 348–57.

77. Wampler, R., Lancisi, D., Indravudh, V., Gautheir, R., and Fine, R., 1999, "A Sealless Centrifugal Blood Pump with Passive Magnetic and Hydrodynamic Bearings," *Artificial Organs* **23**, pp. 780–784, 1999.

78. Slaughter, M. S., Sobieski, M. A., Tamez, D., Horrell, T., Graham, J., Pappas, P. S., Tatooles, A. J., and LaRose, J., 2009, "HeartWrae Miniature Axial Flow Ventricular Assist Device," *Texas Heart Inst. J.*, **36**, pp. 12–16.

79. Jahanmir, S., Hunsberger, A. Z., Heshmat, H., Tomaszewski, M. J., Walton, J. F., Weiss, W. J., Lukic, B., Pae, W. A., Zappanta, C. M., and Khalapyan, T. Z., 2008, "Performance Characterization of MiTiHeart Rotary Centrifugal LVAD with Magnetic Suspension," *Artificial Organs*, **32**, pp. 366–375.

80. Jahanmir, S., Hunsberger, A. Z., Ren, Z., Heshmat, H., Heshmat, C., Tomaszewski, M. J., and Walton, J. F., 2009, "Design of a Small Centrifugal Blood Pump with Magnetic Bearing," *Artificial Organs*, **33**, pp. 714–726.

81. Zhang, Y., Xue, S., Gui, X-M., Sun, H-S., Zhang, H., Zhu, X-D., Hu, S-S., 2007, "A novel Integrated Rotor of Axial Blood Flow Pump Designed with Computational Fluid Dynamics," *Artificial Organs*, **31**(7), pp. 580–575.

82. Qian, K. X., Zeng, P., Ru, W. M., Yuan, H. Y., Feng, Z. G., and Li, L., 2002, "Toward a Durable Impeller Pump with Mechanical Bearings," *ASAIO Journal*, **48**(3), pp. 290–2.

83. Horvath, D. J., Golding, L. A., and Massiello, A., 2001, "The CorAide Blood Pump," *Ann. Thorac. Surg.*, **71**, p. S191.

84. Golding, L. A., Smith, W. A., and Bodmann, D. R., 1996, "The Cleveland Clinic Rotodynamic Pump Program," *Artificial Organs*, **20**(6), pp. 481–4.

85. Fukamachi, K., Horvath, D. J., Massiello, A. L., Ootaki, Y., Kamohara, K., Akiyama, M., Zahr, F., Kopcak, M. W. Jr, Dessoffy, R., Chen, J. F., Benefit, S., and Golding, L. A., 2005, "Development of a Small Implantable Right Ventricular Assist Device," *ASAIO Journal*, **51**(6), pp. 730–5.

86. Chung, M. K. H., Zhang, N., Tansley, G. D., and Woodard, J. C., 2004, "Impeller Behavior and Displacement of the VentrAssist Implantable Rotary Blood Pump," *Artificial Organs*, **28**, pp. 287–297.

87. Vidakovic, S., Ayre, P., Woodard, J. C., Lingard, N., Tansley, G., and Reizes, J., 2000, "Paradoxical Effects of Viscosity on the VentrAssist Rotary Blood Pump," *Artificial Organs*, **24**(6), pp. 478–82.

88. Ayre, P. J., Vidakovic, S. S., Tansley, G. D., Watterson, P. A., and Lovell, N. H., 2000, "Sensorless Flow and Head Estimation in the VentrAssist Rotary Blood Pump," *Artificial Organs*, **24**(8), pp. 585–8.

89. LaRose, J. A., Tamez, D., Ashenuga, M., and Reyes, C., 2010 "Design Concept and Principle of Operation of the HeartWare Ventricular Assist System," *ASAIO Journal*, **56**, pp. 285–289.

90. Tuzun, E., Roberts, K., Cohn, W. E., Sargin, M., Gemmato, C. J., Radovancevic, B., and Frazier, O. H., 2007, "In vivo Evaluation of the HeartWare Centrifugal Ventricular Assist Device," *Texas Heart Inst. J.*, **34**(4), pp. 406–11.

Authors biography

Said Jahanmir is a technology leader with extensive technical and management experience in academia, US government, and industry. He is the President of Boston Tribology Associates, a unique consulting firm providing innovative friction, wear and & lubrication solutions. He has been selected as the ASME Congressional Fellow (2015–2016) and is currently serving as Sr. Legislative Fellow in the Office of Congressman Tim Ryan, providing advice on science and technology, manufacturing, and engineering education. He served as President and CEO of MiTiHeart Corporation and Vice President for biotechnology at Mohawk Innovative Technology, Inc. (2002–2015), where he lead research and development efforts on implantable blood pumps, high-temperature coatings, high-speed micro-machining and high-speed oil-free compressors. His leadership has led to the development and pre-clinical testing of a new generation of mechanical heart assist pumps with magnetic bearings for heart failure patients, and the development of a novel ultra high-speed micro-machining spindle with rotational speeds beyond 500,000 rpm. Prior to joining MiTi he was associated with the National Institute of Standards and Technology (NIST), where he served in several capacities between 1987 and 2002 including Leader of the Ceramic Manufacturing Group. He directed research activities that ranged from characterization of ceramic powders to assessment of mechanical properties of ceramics. He coordinated several international collaborations on pre-standards research that led to ASTM and ISO standards. He established and managed a joint research program between NIST, industry and academia and developed authoritative guides for machining of advanced ceramics. Among his prior experience, he was the first Director of the Tribology Program (1985–87) at the National Science Foundation; Senior Research Engineer (1980–85) at Exxon Research and Engineering Company; Assistant Professor of mechanical engineering (1977–80) at Cornell University; Lecturer (1976–77) at the University of California at Berkeley; and Instructor (1975–76) at the Massachusetts Institute of Technology (MIT). He was an Adjunct Professor of mechanical engineering at the University Delaware (1999–2006) and served as Honorary Research Professor at Hanyang University in South Korea (1998–2002). He has been a

Visiting Lecturer at MIT since 2007 teaching summer short courses in the Professional Education Program.

His pioneering research in tribology, manufacturing and medical devices is widely recognized in the scientific and engineering communities. His groundbreaking research on tribology was instrumental in establishing fundamental mechanics and materials science viewpoint for wear and provided a clear and simple understanding of the fundamentals of boundary lubrication. His research on wear and machining of advanced ceramics and dental materials resulted in a series of highly cited publications. He identified the basic mechanisms of wear and new insights into the fundamental micro-mechanisms of machining and damage formation in advanced ceramics and dental restorations. He has published more than 240 archival papers and major reports and has edited several books and conference proceedings. He has served as the founding Executive Editor of the Machining Science and Technology journal, now in its 18th year. He holds seven US and EU patents.

He received Honorary Membership in ASME in 2013, recognized for seminal contributions to the advancement of mechanical engineering, particularly the multidisciplinary technologies in tribology, manufacturing, biomedical materials and devices, and in the promotion of standards; and for significant contributions to ASME. An ASME Fellow, he has been an active volunteer in the ASME and a strong advocate for change and growth. As chair of the Tribology Division, he revised the bylaws and initiated many innovative projects. Later, as chair of the Board on Research and Technology Development and vice president for research; he streamlined the operating procedures and established fiscal management. As chair of the International Congress Committee he initiated the track-based technical program and encouraged collaboration among ASME divisions and sectors. As a governor at large (2009–12) he served on several Board committees and Presidential task forces, and was a driving force for the ASME Global Impact Strategic Initiative and the new ASME website. He received ASME's Dedicated Service Award in 1995 and Mayo D. Hersey Award in 2001, and the Tribology Division's Donald Wilcock Distinguished Service Award in 2009.

He is a Fellow of the Society of Tribologists and Lubrication Engineers (STLE) and has served in various leadership positions. He is a former member of the American Society for Artificial Internal Organs and the International Society for Rotary Blood Pumps. Among his other honors, Jahanmir received STLE's International Award and Honorary Membership (1997), and the Federal Laboratory Consortium's Technology Transfer Award (2000). He was elected to chair the Gordon Research Conference on Tribology (1998). He served as President of Partnership for Educational Policy (2002–2003), a new organization formed to inform the public and policy makers on educational issues that have a wide reaching impact on K-12 education and was honored as the Community Hero by the Montgomery County Civic Federation (1999) for his contribution to local educational issues. He is listed in Who's Who in America, Who's Who in Science and Engineering and American Men and Women of Science.

He received his bachelor's degree in mechanical engineering from the University of Washington and his master's degree and Ph.D. in mechanical engineering from MIT.

Andrew Hunsberger is a senior engineer at Mohawk Innovative Technology Inc. in Albany, NY, an applied research and product development company specializing in high-speed and extreme environment rotating machinery. Mr. Hunsberger received his B.S. in chemical engineering from Bucknell University in 2001 and M.S. from University of Pittsburgh in bioengineering in 2003.

Mr. Hunsberger has served as MiTi's lead aerodynamic expert for a variety of novel applications including centrifugal hydrogen compressors, micro-turbines and blood pumps. Mr. Hunsberger is involved in a variety of other fields including applied tribology, biocompatible coatings, gas lubricated compliant foil bearings and the application of these technologies to oil-free turbomachinery such as electric motors, turbine engines and fuel cell compressors. Mr. Hunsberger has co-authored over a dozen publications in the fields of hydrogen compressor design, artificial organs, foil bearings and foil seals.

Hooshang Heshmat is a Leading Founder, and President & CEO/ Technical Director of Mohawk Innovative Technology, Inc. (MiTi), an applied research and product development company dedicated to green technology, specializing in advanced rotating machinery development. Since the inception of MiTi in 1994, Dr. Heshmat has directed many new technological advancements specifically targeted toward advanced Oil-Free Rotating Machinery. These advanced machines include:

Synchronous and asynchronous motors/generators with operating speeds from 30,000 to 750,000 rpm and power levels from 200 Watts to 200 kW; High speed fans, blowers and compressors for aircraft cabin environmental control; Industrial and aerospace blower/compressor systems for air, helium, hydrogen and other process gasses in power levels from 1 kW to 200 kW with operating speeds from 360,000 to 60,000 rpm; High-speed, compact, motorized turbo compressors for fuel cell systems (12 to 25 kW); Completely Oil-Free Turbochargers for cars and trucks; Micro/Meso Turbogenerators ranging from 300 Watts to 100 kW, with operating speeds from 500,000 rpm to 30,000 rpm, including an 8 kW/180,000 rpm turbogenerator that produces an equivalent 1 HP/lb; Development of an advanced and novel recuperator system with greater than 90% effectiveness that boosts the 8 kW turbogenerator efficiency from 12 to 28%; Novel, ultra-high-speed micromachining center capable of grinding, milling and drilling at speeds to 500,000 rpm; Left Ventricular Assist Device (LVAD), a unique blood pump with a hybrid bearing system that combines electromagnetic, permanent magnet and hydrodynamic bearings for optimal blood flow conditions and overall patient safety; Developed advance foil bearings and their corresponding coating system that has substantially increased bearing performance capabilities in speed, load carrying capacity, damping, temperature and low ambient pressure conditions. His bearing technology advancements have made it possible to operate his bearing designs in extremely low-ambient pressures, which are enabling development of a new class of advanced flywheels for the energy storage systems. Since the formation of MiTi in 1994, Dr. Heshmat has directed 270 R&D grants/contracts' in the aforementioned technical areas, with an approximate combined value of $75M. He has also nurtured and directed the development of the aforementioned advanced oil free systems, from their concept to fruition, as the Principal Investigator and Team Leader.

Dr. Heshmat and his team of engineers and technologists are specialists in the design and integration of mechanical components (e.g., bearings, seals, dampers and piston rings, including fluid film, dry lubricant and magnetic systems) into Turbomachinery. They are also very experienced in rotating machinery test and measurement techniques, as well as in the design and fabrication of oil-free rotating machinery systems and component test equipment. Dr. Heshmat has established a premier biotechnology company in the Albany, New York area based on their unique heart pump (MiTiHeart).

As a result of his efforts in leading and directing MiTi's technical programs, the company has received the U.S. Small Business Administration's **2002 National Tibbetts Award** in recognition of their outstanding contributions to the SBIR Program, the Albany-Colonie Regional Chamber of Commerce's Small Business Council's **2002 Innovative Enterprise Award** and was listed as the second fastest growing company in the Capital District, the only technology company featured on that top 25 list.

Dr. Heshmat received his B.S. from The Pennsylvania State University in 1977, and his M.S. in 1979 and Ph.D. in 1988 in Mechanical Engineering from Rensselaer Polytechnic Institute. He is the Principal Investigator for a variety of programs concerned with applied tribology, including hydrodynamics, solid lubrication, novel backup bearings for magnetically suspended rotor systems, tribochemistry and surface morphology. Dr. Heshmat's background in tribology encompasses bearings, seals, dampers and piston rings, including both fluid film and dry lubricant systems.

While employed at Reliance Electric Company, Dr. Heshmat was responsible for developing high-performance and cost-effective industrial fluid film bearings ranging from two to 17 inches in diameter. There he developed novel bearings and lubrication systems for starved (partially lubricated) bearings.

Dr. Heshmat has also played a primary role in the development of compliant foil bearings and has been responsible for major advances in this field, including analytical and experimental research for bearing/seal design and application. Much of his work has been related to applying compliant foil bearings to high-speed turbomachinery, including advanced turbine engines (cruise missiles and liquid rocket engines), automotive gas turbines, air-cycle machinery for aircraft, turbochargers, turboexpanders, cryocoolers, pumps, compressors, PM/IM motors and generators, and refrigerant systems. Dr. Heshmat has been investigating the interaction of hybrid foil/magnetic bearings and developed computer codes to permit integrated hybrid bearing designs for advanced gas turbine engine applications.

Dr. Heshmat developed the principle of "Quasi-Hydrodynamic Lubrication with Dry Triboparticulates," i.e., friction and wear control theory for application to extreme environments. This theory was developed based upon his having conducted a wide range of experimental test efforts characterizing fundamental aspects of powder lubrication. Additionally, he has investigated the practical application of this promising new technology to high temperature coatings (Korolon®), dampers and bearings for high-speed gas turbine engines, as well as vacuum environments and damping of structural members, including turbine blades.

Dr. Heshmat is listed in **Who's Who in Business, Who's Who in America** and **Who's Who in the World,** holds 31 patents, has authored more than 185 papers, co-authored 3 chapters (Principles of Bearing Design for the Compressor Handbook, Principles of Gas Turbine Bearing Lubrication and Design for the Theory of Hydrodynamic Lubrication and The Theoretical Analysis of Foil Bearings for the Handbook of Lubrication and Tribology) and authored a book, the **"Tribology of Interface Layers,"** CRC, 2010. He has received the Society of Tribologists and Lubrication Engineers (**STLE) 1983 Wilbur Deutsch Memorial Award,** the American Society of Mechanical Engineers (**ASME) 1985 Burt L. Newkirk Award,** the Mechanical Technology Incorporated (MTI) 1990 Technical **Creativity Award** for his pioneering work in powder lubrication and the **STLE 1993 Captain Alfred E. Hunt Award** for the best paper published by the society, "The Quasi-Hydrodynamic Mechanism of Powder Lubrication: Part II - Lubricant Film Pressure Profile." He is an active member of STLE/ASME, was Chairman of the 1994 International Joint ASME/STLE Tribology Conference, Chairman of the Research Committee on Tribology of ASME (1999–2000), a member of the ASME Tribology Division Honors and Awards and Executive Committees, an invited speaker for the January 1997 ASME Satellite Broadcast on The Selection, Design, and Performance of Bearings and Seals and was promoted to the grade of **ASME & STLE Fellow** in 1998. For his pioneering work in the field of compliant surface hydrodynamic foil bearings, he received the prestigious **ASME/RCT 1995 Creative Research Award.** He was the recipient of **STLE's 1996 Al Sonntag Award** for the outstanding paper written on solid lubrication and published in the society journal, "The Quasi-Hydrodynamic Mechanism of Powder Lubrication: Part III - On Theory and Rheology of Triboparticulates," and **ASME/IGTI 1999 Best Paper Award,** "Application of Foil Bearings to Turbomachinery

Including Vertical Operation". He was chosen to receive the ASME Board on Research and Technology Development's **2002 Thomas A. Edison Patent Award** and STLE **2003 Frank P. Bussick Award** for authoring the best paper on Sealing Systems Technology, "Performance of a Compliant Foil Seal in a Small Gas Turbine Engine Simulator Employing a Hybrid Foil/Ball Bearing Support System," published by the Society. Dr. Heshmat also received the ASME IGTI **2005 Microturbine and Small Turbomachinery Committee Best Paper Award** for authoring "Demonstration of a Turbojet Engine Using an Air Foil Bearing," ASME Paper GT2005-68404, the ASME **2007 Mayo D. Hersey** award for significant contributions to the fundamental science of powder lubrication and advanced compliant foil bearings and the STLE **2008 International Award** in recognition of his outstanding contribution to the field of tribology and entitling him to a lifetime membership in the STLE. Dr. Heshmat was also presented the Pennsylvania State University **2009 Alumni Achievement Award** for his extraordinary professional accomplishments and the ASME **2009 Propulsion Best Paper Award** for his technical paper entitled "Innovative High Temperature Compliant Surface Foil Face Seal Development," the **Japanese Society of Tribologists 2014 Best Paper Award** for the technical paper "Oil-Free Bearings and Seals for Centrifugal Hydrogen Compressor" and the **ASME IGIT 2014 Best Paper Award** for "Oil-Free 8 kW High-Speed and High Specific Power Turbogenerator." In 2016, Dr. Heshmat became a member of the **LaMCoS/INSA Lyon International Advisory Board** (IAB). For more information, please visit our home page at: http://www.miti.cc or http://www.heshmat.cc.